Across the Chasm: A Caregiver's Story

By Naomi L. Zikmund-Fisher
with Brian J. Zikmund-Fisher

bmt *infonet*
BLOOD & MARROW TRANSPLANT
INFORMATION NETWORK
2310 Skokie Valley Road • Suite 104
Highland Park • Illinois 60035 USA

phone 847.433.3313
fax 847.433.4599
toll-free 888.597.7674

e-mail help@bmtnews.org
website http://www.bmtnews.org

For Aaron, Cliff, Cyndi,
Jessie, Sharon, Suzanne,
and all the other caregivers
who cross the chasm every day

Acknowledgements

I should say, before you read any further, that I never set out to write a book. What you hold in your hands is a carefully edited catharsis, nothing more. The messages which form the basis for this book were sent over the course of two and a half years to an electronic mailing list of about 60 friends and family. The majority of them also appeared on the Internet mailing list BMT-talk, maintained by the Association of Cancer Online Resources (ACOR). They have been edited, and I have added in thoughts that I didn't feel I could share at the time the messages were originally written. I have tried very hard to maintain the spontaneous narratives and emotions which formed the soul of the caregiving experience for me. In some places, where I added in events that I had not originally chronicled, I may have missed the actual dates on which they occurred by a few days. I apologize.

A book such as this one really requires two sets of acknowledgements-- one for the people who made the book possible, and one for the people who made the experience upon which the book is based possible.

I would like to thank my parents, Franklin and Ellen Fisher, for insisting that my writing should be published even when I wasn't very sure. I would also like to thank Carol Fradkin at BMT InfoNet for being the first person outside my immediate circle who thought it was worth reading, cover to cover, and for passing it on, as well as for her comments on previous drafts of the manuscript. My deepest appreciation to Susan Stewart of BMT InfoNet for extensive comments and suggestions, as well as for having the vision to see a need for a book about caregiving and helping to make it happen. Brian Zikmund-Fisher also provided editorial comment, which, although I didn't always want to hear it, was enormously helpful in shaping the book. Shirley Beltz donated her time and talent to design the cover.

I would like to thank ACOR for providing a forum where I could write in the first place. I am extremely grateful to my friends and family, as well as the more than 1,200 people who read BMT-talk, for providing me an audience. Had I not known there were people reading, this writing would not have happened.

The experience upon which this book is based was the most difficult of my life. Without the help and support of literally hundreds of people, I could not have made it through.

I would like to acknowledge, first and foremost, the staff of Brian's transplant center. The expertise, care and dedication of these men and women made this experience so much easier for both of us. I would like to specifically mention Pat Groff, Eileen Cruse, Andi Bowen, Moreen Shannon-Dudley and Chuck the receptionist, all of whom kept me sane and my husband healthy. Thanks also to Eduardo Benedetti, Julian Sevilla, Patricia Stewart and James Wade for their incredible care.

At home, Brian and I have been blessed with a medical team that often crosses the line between professional care and personal friendship. Delynne Myers, William Mitsos and Lane Linden made everything in this book possible, and more.

The support of friends and family was invaluable in getting us through. Mark Miller gave up his personal life for four months to support us. Barbara and Joseph Zikmund gave up their lives entirely to make this work.

Our "home team" made sure that we were not forgotten, and we are forever grateful. Michelle Katz, lawyer, friend and godmother extraordinaire and Nancy Dubuar, the phone-call lady and wonderful friend, deserve special mentions. Thanks also to Eleanor Lewis and Elizabeth McGuire, who made us feel like heroes every step of the way. My appreciation to Abigail Fisher, Abraham Fisher and Colleen Humphreys for all their love and support, and to their children, Beth, Wendy, Jamie, Teddy, Valerie and Harry for their gifts of artwork and love.

There are many, many others, too many to name, who lent their heart and soul to making sure the Zikmund-Fishers got to transplant and back in one piece. We can never repay the debt of gratitude we owe you.

And, of course, we are forever grateful to Australian Bone Marrow Donor Registry donor number 4021-4102-2 for his totally selfless gift of life.

Lastly, I would like to thank my wonderful husband, Brian, and my fantastic daughter, Eve Joelle, for making the chasm worth crossing. For you, I'd do it again.

Naomi Zikmund-Fisher
April 27, 2001

Foreword

"The whole world is a very narrow bridge,
And the most important thing is not to be afraid."
—Rabbi Nachman of Bratslav

Some messages are impossible to say "right." This is one of them.

As a few of you know, I have a history of difficulties with my blood, back when I was a teenager. These problems appeared to have resolved themselves. Until now.

I have been diagnosed with myelodysplastic syndrome (MDS), a progressive dysfunction of the bone marrow which, in my case, has dropped my platelet count (remember platelets, those cute things which start the clotting process??) to dangerous levels and has begun to affect production of other blood cells as well. MDS is only treatable in symptoms. One can transfuse platelets or blood, and there are some medications which may support the blood counts in the short run, but one cannot fix the underlying problem. One can, however, replace it.

As you read this on Tuesday, I will be at an intake appointment to a bone marrow transplant program. Since I have no siblings and other family are unlikely to be matches, they will begin the process of searching for an unrelated marrow donor and discuss the implications of this truly terrifying procedure.

The good news, such as there is, is that MDS patients whose transplants are successful are quite likely to live long-term and disease free. The relapse rate for MDS in the refractive anemia (RA) stage, which is where I am, is lower than for some other diagnoses.

The bad news is that, any time you use chemotherapy to wipe out one's immune system, even a minor cold can kill you and, unfortunately, sometimes it does. In addition, I'll have to take drugs to suppress my immune system after the new one grows in, so I'll still be vulnerable. And we have to hope that the chemo and the transplant don't cause other problems. The procedure takes months to years of time, both in and out of the hospital, and is not, shall we say, painless. I've been given about a 25% chance of not making it through the first year. But, unless we can arrest the changes in my marrow, which is unlikely, my chances without transplant are much worse.

Seem out of the blue? Think you've been hallucinating since you've seen me running across campus recently? You're not going insane. Fortunately, through all this, I feel fine. Too fine, if anything. And thus, I continue to do my work, to live my life to the fullest extent possible and do pretty much what I want. Naomi and I are looking forward to the birth of our first child in May, and we refuse to let this completely overshadow our joy in that. As frustrating as this all is, I take that gift and value it.

Why am I telling you all this, and why now? Two reasons:

1) I don't want to pretend any more that I'm "OK" when I am definitely not OK. I want to be able to talk about what's going on without being afraid of how to broach the subject in the first place. And, on the good side, I'm tired of pretending that I should be "strong" and deal with this alone when I know (though sometimes I forget) that I have a ton of friends and colleagues who can help me and Naomi through this. I'm not going to be afraid anymore to welcome that help.

2) I want to ask each of you to consider being typed as a bone marrow donor in the National Marrow Donor Program registry. A perfect match can be really hard to find. All too often a transplant never happens because no one can be found who can serve as a donor.

As I sit here today, I will not know for weeks whether a match can be found for me or not. It seems so ridiculous to me that anyone should face such uncertainty. I will have to rely on the probabilities that someone matching me has chosen to be typed and to be in the registry without ever knowing if they would be needed. I want to live in a world where anyone needing such a transplant can reasonably expect to find a donor. Do not get typed just for me — the likelihood of a match is miniscule. If you want to do anything at all for me, get typed for everyone.

How can you get typed?

Well, for those of you in Pittsburgh, the Central Blood bank will do the typing. Contact their central office for information. The next blood drive at Carnegie Mellon University will also be a typing drive, but don't feel you need to wait until then.

For those of you not in Pittsburgh, call 1-800-MARROW2 for the number of the nearest NMDP donor center to you. I have a list of all of the typing centers in the country myself, so you can also e-mail me and I'll give you the info for centers near you.

What does all this mean?

It means I cannot say with any certainty whether I will be around the university much over the next year. It means that if I need this procedure, which is not certain but seems more and more likely, I will be sidelined for quite some time. Nothing will happen for a couple of months, that much seems certain. Beyond that, however, is anyone's guess.

I don't quite know how to end this note, so I guess it'll just end. Thanks.

Brian

Date: Fri, 5 Jun 1998
From: Brian J Zikmund-Fisher
Subject: Eve Joelle Zikmund-Fisher

Family and Friends,

     Naomi and I are both pleased and amazed to announce the birth of our daughter, Eve Joelle Zikmund-Fisher, who came into our arms at 5:04AM on Friday, June 5. Eve weighed 7 lbs., 12 oz., was 19 inches long, has a mess-load of dark hair already and appears to be quite healthy.

     The naming ceremony to honor Eve will be held at 5:00 PM, Friday, June 12 at our home.

Brian

Across the Chasm

"You can't cross a chasm in two small jumps."
—David Lloyd George

Chapter 1:
The Search

Date: Wed, 9 Dec 1998
From: Naomi L Zikmund-Fisher
Subject: Update on Brian (long)

First off, I'd like to welcome those of you new to THE LIST, an electronic mailing list that is growing at quite a clip. Brian has asked me to add various people from here on in, including his doctors and some assorted other miscreants. If you have not been receiving these updates until now it's because a) I didn't have your address, b) I forgot about you, c) Brian has been keeping you apprised on his own or d) all of the above. Please don't take it personally, and welcome to our happy little family of people who are somehow or another touched by Brian's health situation.

When we last left our hero, he had decided to travel across the country for his bone marrow transplant to treat the MDS which has decimated his blood counts and left him transfusion dependent for platelets. His donor search had been started here in Pittsburgh, so he needed to officially transfer responsibility for finding a donor from here to the new center. We filled out the forms to change our insurance, since our old plan wouldn't cover the transplant if he had it out of the region.

The decision to do this was incredibly hard. On the one hand, there was the daunting prospect of leaving our support system thousands of miles away, traveling with an infant, setting up in a new place where we knew no one for four or more months and all that good stuff. On the other hand, our consult at this transplant center convinced us that these people really know what they're doing and have experience with patients like Brian. And, frankly, I'm not ready to be a widow and single mother at age 28 and he's not ready to die at age 29. Picky us.

After an arduous week of discussion between our return from the consult and the day the insurance open-enrollment forms were due, Brian made the choice. Then, of course, we had to figure out, to the penny, which of my employer's health plans made the most sense for this situation. But that's another story. Everyone seems to have an opinion about whether the choice to go out of town is the right one, but, frankly, we don't want to hear it. This is stressful enough without the second-guessing and the I-told-you-so's.

Since then, many of you have asked the obvious question, "Now what." We find ourselves asking this, too, with some frequency.

As we speak, the folks at the lab are re-testing Brian's bone marrow type and we are awaiting with baited breath the arrival of blood samples from four potential donors. Three of these donors were identified here as matches for Brian, and one looks promising. Brian and all of his donors must be retyped for two reasons. First of all, a mistake in the typing could be catastrophic for Brian. Second of all, each center has its own criteria for choosing suitable donors, so this lab wants some different information about people's typing than was previously done.

Meanwhile, Brian's parents are also being typed again. Although we know from previous testing that they are not suitable matches for him, having them typed serves as an extra check that Brian's typing was done correctly. Because Brian gets half of his marrow type from each of his parents, the lab can double check that those halves do indeed come up as matches. If they don't, they know that someone's typing was done wrong.

Anyway, all of the retyping of Brian and his donors should take another three or so weeks. With any luck, a donor will be found from the four in question. If not, there are many others to try. These were just the most promising. With luck, we could be leaving roughly the last week in January or perhaps the beginning of February.

Brian will soon be going *in absentia* from his graduate program at Carnegie Mellon University. As most of you know, he's getting his doctorate in Social and Decision Sciences. It seems kind of ironic to be putting all that information about decision making to such practical use. Brian will not officially be going to school in the months ahead. Since he's working on his dissertation right now, however, he can continue to work on it even after the university thinks he's off under some rock somewhere.

I am still on maternity leave from my elementary special education teaching position with the Pittsburgh Public Schools, and I'm extending that for "personal reasons." The Board of Education has been very nice about this, thank God. So we have the flexibility to do what we need to do, and, since I wasn't planning on working now anyway and Brian doesn't earn all that much, we're financially prepared as well.

We have tentatively arranged for a couple whom we met through a woman in my playgroup to live in our house while we are away. They are looking for a month-to-month rental, we are looking for someone to keep the burglars away, so it works out. However, this is still tentative, so if you know anyone who wants to not sublet our house (because that would be against the lease, of course) on a very transient and indefinite basis starting sometime, but we're not sure when, let us know. We have arranged for our next door neighbors to take in our cat, Gul du Cat, as a foster kitty while we're gone.

We will be renting an apartment near the transplant center — there are several buildings that cater largely to patients and their families. Brian's parents and my parents are all planning on coming out to help us for large chunks of time. Brian will be outpatient for two weeks before transplant, inpatient for one week before transplant, inpatient for anywhere from three weeks to two months after transplant and then outpatient thereafter. There's always the possibility, of course, that he will need to be readmitted. But we can't do anything about that, so it seems better to just keep our eyes on the best case scenario for now.

10

We will probably be away for roughly three months after transplant, total. So, for you math mavens, that's three months and three weeks out of town, give or take a humongous margin of error.

Meanwhile, while the lab does the typing, we just wait. We are not good at waiting. We hate waiting. Waiting is amazingly stressful. Brian is currently receiving platelet transfusions about every 8-10 days and getting periodic blood tests. Other than that, we wait. Wait wait wait. We are still hoping to go to New England from the 20th to the 27th for our families' Chanumas celebrations. Or is that Christuka? Who said inter-faith marriage was easy? That should at least vary the waiting some.

Many of you have asked what you can do. At the moment, we ask just a few favors:

First, keep those calls and e-mails coming. A lot of people have said, "I was going to call, but I know you must be bombarded." We like being bombarded. Bombarded is good. Yes, we are under a lot of stress, but the best way we know to relieve it is to have contact with our friends (OK, that and hot fudge. Hot fudge with friends is even better). We're trying to live as normal lives as humanly possible right now. It's hard. We find ourselves pouncing on other people's problems to try to solve them because we can't solve our own, and it makes us feel like we're doing something. So now is a really good time to tell us your troubles. We'll try to solve them over hot fudge.

Second, if you haven't gotten the noodgy message yet, go get typed as a bone marrow donor. If you've been typed, let us know. It really lifts our spirits because, again, it makes us feel like we've done something. I subscribe to an Internet list about BMT and a lot of people are not nearly as lucky as Brian in finding a donor. You are needed.

Third, go give blood. Right now, Brian is getting platelets from a single, directed, very kind donor. This woman is someone we've never met who heard about Brian and wanted to help. So he doesn't actually physically need your platelets. However, there are plenty of people out there who do. The volume of platelets a patient like Brian gets is ordinarily spun from six units of whole blood. That means that six people need to give blood for each time a patient gets a platelet transfusion. You are needed this way, too. If you're up to the challenge, you can also become a platelet donor by calling your local blood bank. You can really make a difference. And, again, if you've done this due to our noodging, please let us know.

This concludes the Public Service Announcement portion of this message. Thanks to all for your caring and concern. We'll be in touch with more news soon!

A joyous Chanumas to all!

naomi

Date: Wed, 30 Dec 1998
Subject: Good news and bad news

We have good news and bad news. For a change, we're going to start with the bad news because it puts the good news in some context.

As you know, the transplant center is searching for a MUD (that's matched unrelated donor, not moistened soil) for Brian. They requested confirmatory typing on three donors who were previously found to be perfect matches for him, as well as one additional donor. This week, we received word that the first three of these four donors are mismatched with Brian on HLA-C, an antigen that had not previously been typed. It seems that roughly 50% of people with Brian's other antigens match his HLA-C, so you would think that, out of three donors, at least one would be a match. Well, you would be wrong. We're awaiting word on the fourth donor.

Now, don't get too upset yet because 1) There are still 53 (yes you read that correctly) known 6/6 matches in the registry whom they haven't even requested confirmatory samples from, 2) there are an additional 800 or so 4/4 matches whom we could start typing if we really needed to and 3) the docs are pretty vague about how much HLA-C actually matters in the outcome of the transplant, so if worst comes to worst they could use any one of these three donors.

So the current plan is to request a mess more donor samples and see who comes out as a good match. This will take some more time — probably three or more weeks — but is not the end of the world, except as it affects the "waiting" factor which you know we all love.

OK, on to the good news.

Brian returned from vacation on Sunday and, on Monday, dutifully reported for his blood test and (we thought) platelet transfusion. Much to our surprise, however, his counts were all up from his last test 11 days before. His platelet count had doubled from the last untransfused number we had, his red cells were up, his white cells were up. Very strange. So he forewent the transfusion on Monday and went back today for another test. We really expected all his numbers to be back down. However, today his platelets were up ever so slightly again and his red counts were up quite a bit. His platelets are at a level we haven't seen without transfusion in several months. His red counts were last this high at the end of October.

Now, to put this in perspective, if you or I went to the doctor for a physical and had a blood test done and came up with these numbers, we would be setting off all kinds of alarm bells and getting panicked phone calls from our doctors demanding that we get ourselves to a hematologist post haste. I don't in any way want to give the impression that Brian is somehow "better." But the numbers are better than they were, which, in a disease that one expects to get worse at a steady pace, is a little unexpected.

What does this mean? We sure have no idea. In the short run it means no transfusion for a while. In the long run, we have no expectation that

12

his numbers will stay at the level where they are now, let alone continue up. But any week without a transfusion is good, and it takes a little bit of the donor search time pressure off since, for at least a short while, he isn't transfusion dependent. You see, over time the body sensitizes to transfusions, making the transplant harder because it's harder to get blood products the body will accept, so fewer transfusions is better.

It's hard not to get hopeful with the counts looking up. We know they'll be looking down again, but somehow we don't want to acknowledge that. For nine months we've been saying, "I'm ready to wake up from the nightmare now," so it's hard not to feel like the alarm on the clock radio is about to go off, even though we know in our hearts that that isn't going to happen.

Meanwhile, we recently executed new wills, powers of attorney and living wills. We're revisiting our ancient conflict over the fact that Brian doesn't believe in burial and I don't believe in cremation. And, of course, even if I were to bury Brian I'm not sure where that would be. Brian's parents suggested the town where he was born, but that seems to negate the fact that he has a life past childhood, somehow. We're leaning toward either a really pretty cemetery near my parent's house or the cemetery our congregation uses here. We've also discussed how long I would keep our hyphenated name if he were to die and how long I would wear my wedding ring. Brian says I should give myself permission to not know the answers to those questions. That's hard to do. We've also talked about what I should tell Eve about her Daddy, which is the hardest thing of all to discuss.

All of this may sound morbid. I know everyone thinks we should be "full speed ahead, chin up, don't look down" about this. But, believe it or not, dealing with this stuff now helps us cope with the fact that it exists at all. Not dealing with it makes me worry more about it because I know I'll have to deal with it if Brian dies, and I'll feel less able to cope then. Dealing with the prospect that Brian might die helps us put it to the side and move on with the prospect that Brian might live. I don't know if you can understand that unless you've faced this kind of situation yourself.

So, to summarize, we don't know when we're leaving and won't for awhile. We'll let you know, don't worry, so please don't ask! In the meantime, Brian gets a break from transfusions, which is nice because he is getting kind of tired of me and the nurses in the treatment room teasing him about what a weenie he is about IV's.

So, we continue to wait and wait and wait. The hot fudge is gravitating to our hips but is much appreciated, as are all your prayers, thoughts, calls, letters, smoke signals, etc. We're keeping busy running around trying to get every conceivable piece of medical care we possibly can before we leave our HMO tomorrow for the "traditional" health plan that will cover Brian's transplant. And then, of course, tomorrow night we're gonna party like it's 1999.

Happy new year to one and all, and best of luck remembering to date your checks properly come Friday.

naomi

We've been putting off sending this latest e-mail until we had something definitive to say. We have come to the startling conclusion, however, that that's going to be a while, so we either need to send it out anyway or stop answering our phone. As the latter would kill us, here's the latest on Brian . . .

We got a call last week saying that the transplant center felt it would be OK to proceed with one of the donors who had already been typed. This is a young, "big," cytomegalovirus (CMV) negative, ABO compatible male. Young donors are preferable, as are "gender matched" donors. CMV is a virus that about 50% of the population has been exposed to but Brian hasn't, and we'd like to keep it that way. ABO is blood type — you can do a transplant with a mismatch but it's nice if you don't have to. "Big" donors are good for "big" patients because they have a better shot at getting enough cells from the donor.

The only catch about this donor is that he is a mismatch on one HLA-C antigen. Although not one of the antigens usually discussed when we talk about "4 of 4" and "6 of 6" matches, HLA-C has been shown to substantially affect the rate of graft failure (the new marrow not "taking") in patients with chronic myelogenous leukemia (CML). Now, Brian doesn't have CML, but they don't know whether the same would be true for MDS patients.

So, to cut through the techy stuff, this donor is good but not perfect. But the transplant center felt it might be better to go ahead with this one anyway because they don't want Brian to get a lot more transfusions before his transplant. The benefit of this donor seemed like it might outweigh the risk, but it was a judgement call.

So, based on this donor, we were given an arrival date of February 24 with a tentative transplant date around the 17th of March. We were going to inquire whether they could dye the marrow green. We had very mixed feelings about going ahead with this, both because of the mismatch and because this meant we were actually going to have to do this, and, frankly, we aren't terribly enthused about it even though we know it's inevitable. Still, we started to make some plans and booked an apartment. We were waiting to speak with a doctor who is something of an expert on HLA-C mismatches before we sent out the final word that we were leaving.

In the meantime, Brian went in on Tuesday for his weekly blood test to discover that his counts have risen again. He has not had a transfusion since December 18 and things are going up, much to everyone's surprise. His platelet count in particular is still alarmingly low, but it's more than twice what it was at the beginning of December. On the other hand, two times zero is still zero. To cut to the chase, Brian has decided, after talking to his hematologist here and to the folks at the transplant center, that if his counts stay where they are or go up some more, he is waiting for a better-matched donor if one can be found. If his counts head south again, he'll go with the one he has. We are keeping the date for the 24th for the time being because 1) his counts could be back in the sewer next week and 2) if a better-matched donor is found in the next couple of weeks we can still keep that schedule.

I want to make a couple of things really clear. First, Brian is not "cured" by any stretch of the imagination. The only cure for MDS is the transplant. But something vaguely positive is obviously going on. Second, Brian will, in the future, have a bone marrow transplant. It's hard to know when, and sooner is much more likely than later, but it is going to happen. We may not like that truth, but it's there.

At the risk of sounding flaky, it feels like this whole situation is a sign. We've spent so much time worrying that Brian might not make it through this. And suddenly, when he needs it most, his counts start going up. I just have to believe that God isn't ready for Brian to die, at least not yet. Let's hope God continues to feel that way.

In other news, some of you might think that I am taking the opportunity presented by my maternity/family emergency leave to relax. Ha. My teaching job is fast being replaced with my full-time occupation of writing angry letters and yelling over the phone to our health insurance company. The company seems to have restructured into a format whereby decisions are made by poltergeists who immediately disappear into the ether, leaving only computer notations, which are read to me by people with no power to change anything. Their new corporate motto is, "If we're wrong, you can't do a damned thing about it."

They have denied coverage for Brian's donor search. They told me that it's (I'm not making this up) "excluded because it's not included." When I appealed, they then denied that I even have the right to appeal it. I had to fax them the section of my benefits book entitled "Appeal Process" to convince them otherwise. I've gotten the folks at the Office of Patient Advocacy at the National Marrow Donor Program involved in helping me navigate the mess, and they've told me I'm "very good at this," confirming my belief that my true calling in life is not in the classroom, but rather knocking heads.

Every stage of this fiasco requires at least two hours of telephone calls, at least 90 minutes of which is spent on hold. And that's in addition to the time I spend filling out claim forms for Brian's medications and all that fun stuff. I've hired my best friend, Michelle, godmother of my child and mother of my goddaughter, as our lawyer in this matter. If she can't do it, I'm not sure who can.

So, that's what's new here. As we keep saying, we'll let you know what we know. We thank you all for your continued support. Watch this space for further updates.

Oh, and when was the last time you gave blood?

naomi

Date: Tue, 2 Feb 1999
Subject: Victory!

Just wanted to share our most excellent news. After much phone calling, letter writing, involvement of the NMDP and my employer and able legal advice from Michelle, Blue Cross and Blue Shield called today to say:

"Mass screening and testing may also be included in the donor search."

This means that they at least theoretically will now cover Brian's ever lengthening search for an unrelated donor. Without quoting actual numbers, let's just say this is a victory well into five figures. I am feeling a little proud of myself, although now I'll have to find a new hobby.

And now, in Michelle's honor, I have to go out and find Eve a T-shirt that says, "My godmother can beat up your godmother."

naomi

Date: Tue, 9 Feb 1999
Subject: no news is no news

Time for another one of those wacky updates from Naomi about Brian!

When we last left our hero, counts were stable and spirits were good and we weren't really sure what we were doing. This week on "The Young and the Myelodysplastic" . . .

Brian's counts continue to be pretty good. His red counts are now in the normal range, his whites are meandering their way up, and platelets are holding the line at the "alarming but not transfusion dependent" level.

Brian had a bone marrow biopsy last Thursday — his fifth overall and his third this year. These are, as I gather it, extremely unpleasant. They certainly look it to the concerned spouse. During the one before this one I had to suppress the urge to clock the nurse practitioner who was doing it. At any rate, the news from this latest one is that the marrow looks "a *bit* better" (emphasis his hematologist's, not mine) and there are a few more normal cells, but this might just be a sampling error. It's not a major change. No surprise. The good news is that the blast count is still around 0%. Blasts are bad — they're what the marrow produces when you have leukemia.

On the donor front, they have now come up with a donor who is fully matched with him on all of the antigens they test for. However, this person is a different blood type (not a very big deal) and CMV+ (potentially a bigger deal, or at least we'd like to avoid it). This donor is the best thus far, but we're still looking, and given Brian's general stability (physical at least) we have time to look.

Soooo, the long and the short of it is, we have canceled our date for February 24. The time for transplant is coming, sooner and not later, but it's not here, at least not until he has a better donor. Samples are pouring in as we speak from potential other donors (and, may I add gloatingly, at no cost to us!!!!), and we hope to know more soon.

Thanks once again for all your support. We'll be in touch, watch this space.

naomi

Date: Sat, 27 Feb 1999
Subject: More absence of news

This is a non-update. It's been almost 3 weeks since last I wrote, and I therefore feel I ought to let you know what's happening, but the real answer is, "not much."

Brian's counts started to come back down two weeks ago. He had a horrible cold at the time and wound up with a nosebleed that pretty much wouldn't stop, so he had a platelet transfusion even though his counts were not at the level where he usually needs one. Frankly, he just freaked out about the nosebleed, and the transfusion was more to put his mind at ease than anything else. Monday will be his first "unsupported" blood test (where the transfusion isn't bumping up his count) since that transfusion, and we'll see.

The donor we thought we had — fully matched but ABO mismatched and CMV+ — turns out to be a molecular mismatch at HLA-A. For those of you not experienced with this stuff, don't worry about what that means. Suffice to say that he looked like a full match but more complex testing revealed that he wasn't.

So, on goes the search. There are still umpteen people (umpteen being the technical, medical term) with samples at the lab whose typing isn't yet completed, and we expect those to be done in the next three weeks or so. Then one of these lucky folks will be chosen as Brian's donor.

Many of our friends and family have commented that we've been less communicative about our plans recently. This is undoubtedly true. I guess we're tired of announcing plans that get changed and then having to explain everything all over again. We're feeling a little noodged by people who keep asking what's going on. It's not like we'd keep it a secret if they ever found Brian a donor! We're not trying to be evasive or secretive. We're just trying to maintain our personal space and cut down on the number of people we have to keep updated on a minute-to-minute basis.

That doesn't mean you shouldn't call. We appreciate your company. It does mean, however, that you probably shouldn't call, ask if they've found a donor yet, and then hang up. At least not if you want to live.

Meanwhile, back at the ranch:

Our insurance company, which, on February 2, called to say they would be covering Brian's search, called on the 11th to say they were "investigating" this. On the 12th, they faxed a copy of an internal memo (that is, a memo written from one of their departments to another) to the transplant center which, in essence, said, "I don't care if you want to cover this or not. You told her you would and now you have to." Then, this Monday, they called and said they would cover it as it is being billed now, but if it were billed under other codes we were out of luck, because "mass screening isn't covered." I actually had to fax their own memo back to them. For those of you keeping score, that's a total of

18

four total or partial mind changes in less than a month.

So, at present, we think we have coverage but we can't get them to admit it. When I pointed out that they are required to respond to our appeal within 30 days in writing and it was 46 days and still nothing in writing, the woman actually said, "I'm corresponding with you by phone." So, our incredibly able attorney Michelle is making some more calls, and we've filed a complaint with the insurance commission.

Truth told, I'm now finding this downright entertaining, and it keeps me busy. I have great faith that our bills will be paid and no faith that it will be easy from here on in. I'm just rolling with it.

That's the news from here. Thanks to one and all for your prayers, support, and, of course, hot fudge (frankly, we should have thought of that angle sooner!). Thanks also to those who have called and written to say, "I hope you're happy, you made me feel so guilty that I became a marrow donor (or gave blood, as the case may be)." Guilt is a powerful tool, and we are honored that you have allowed us to wield it in your direction for this worthy cause.

More news as it happens. Watch this space.

naomi

OK, so, what's new? You ask.
Nothing.
Well, that's not really totally true, but the bottom line is:
Nothing.

The lab is now down to the last three (3) (trois) (shalosh) (eethray) possible candidates for Brian's donor without going into the 800 or so people who are known to match him on the first four antigens but about whom we know nothing else. One of this aforementioned troika is a full serologic match for Brian, and we're awaiting the high-resolution DNA results. The other two are still pending. We expect the DNA on the first one in about 11 days, DNA if we need it on the other two around then as well, and then, God willing, we will be scheduling.

We have pretty much given up on trying to give definite ideas about when we will be leaving, and resigned ourselves to the fact that we have absolutely no control over this. This is really hard for us, since, as you are well aware, we are major control freaks.

I continue to keep myself busy filling out claim forms, obsessing about insurance, and bugging the heck out of my fabulous attorney. She actually had us come visit her in State College, PA last weekend so I would stop calling every three minutes, if only for two days. We have decided that the insurance company is processing our claims using a magic 8-ball: Is this covered? "Answer hazy, try again later."

The insurance company finally determined in writing that they would cover the testing for the three weeks in February when they said they would, but not the rest. However, they then started paying some of the charges from other days, all the while yelling that they wouldn't and that they couldn't understand why we didn't grasp that. This seemingly random interaction with customer service does not generally aid our feeling of absence of control, shall we say.

So, you remember in Psych 101, that experiment with the dogs where they taught them to jump over a barrier to avoid an electric shock? They then discovered you could induce depression by shocking them even when they jumped over the barrier so they couldn't avoid the shock no matter what they did. Well, we feel like we're in the middle of that experiment. We have learned helplessness, and it ain't much fun.

Although we have no news, we still live day to day with the stress of the situation and with the enormity of what lies ahead, and it gets to us. Which is a fancy way of saying, just because when you call we don't have news doesn't mean you shouldn't call. We're not avoiding you; we just don't have much to add. And frankly, we can use the diversion your company provides. We need to know our friends are still out there.

Today marks the one-year anniversary of my last day of work. One year ago today I was in pre-term labor. Come to think of it, do you think that the stress of having a husband diagnosed with a life threatening illness less than two weeks before could have had anything to do with that? Nah.

Anyway, this time last year I was counting contractions and praying that Consuela (which is what we called Eve before we knew she was Eve) wouldn't arrive too soon. Now I just pray I won't find cheerios between her toes when I take off her socks. A lot can happen in a year. We're just glad to have spent it together, and hoping and praying to do the same with the next one.

So, that's what's new here. Nothing.
Watch this space.

naomi

Date: Thu, 25 Mar 1999
Subject: A chance to do some good

In Judaism, as in many other traditions, it is customary to make a gift to *tzedakah*, (charity) when one prays for the healing of a loved one. Over the last several months, a number of you have inquired as to where might be an appropriate place to send tzedakah for Brian's speedy recovery.

Brian and I are pleased to announce that we have set up a fund in Brian's honor at the HLA Registry Foundation. HLA Registry is the largest bone marrow donor recruitment center in the country, with over 160,000 donors under their purview. Donations made in honor of Brian will be used to fund DR typing on new and existing donors. This will help to make the search for a bone marrow donor faster, more effective, and cheaper for patients, who are often quite short on time and, unfortunately, insurance for their search. For those of you not familiar with bone marrow typing, see my explanation of what this is and why it's important below.

Donations may be sent to:

HLA Registry Foundation, Inc.
70 Grand Avenue
River Edge, NJ 07661
Attn: Brian Zikmund-Fisher Fund

Make the check out to HLA Registry Foundation, Inc. Be sure to indicate Brian Zikmund-Fisher Fund on your check or in your letter, so 1) your money will go toward DR typing and 2) we can write you a nice thank you note. Of course, you don't need to do this in honor of Brian (Flag Day is just around the corner, for example), and you certainly don't need to be Jewish! But we hope you will help. Feel free to print this out and save it for end-of-year charitable giving. Donations to HLA Registry are tax deductible.

We thank all of you for your continued prayers and support. We hope to have a final departure date sometime next week, and we'll let you know as soon as we do.

naomi

DR Typing and Why It's Important
(I thought "DR Typing for Dummies" was unnecessarily mean):

Frequently, when people are typed as bone marrow donors, they are typed at four antigens: two at HLA-A and two at HLA-B. This goes into the computer and is available to hospitals conducting donor searches for patients. However, there are really many more criteria for matching a donor with a patient. The next two antigens generally tested are two antigens at DR. When

22

patients talk about finding a "six of six match," they mean the donor matches at A, B and DR. If you are a registered donor and you are called for more testing, the first thing they are likely to test for is DR, and that information goes into the computer, too.

At this point, about 44% of donors in the National Marrow Donor Program (NMDP) are already typed at DR, and that information is available for searches. The trouble is, the NMDP has gotten sufficiently big that it is like looking for a needle in a haystack to try to find someone who is a perfect match by typing all the people who are only known to match a patient at A and B. Recording donors by A and B is simply not enough information anymore. More donors of the remaining 56% need to be typed at DR.

For example, for Brian, there were 58 six of six matches in the registry, but over 800 four of fours, that is, people who matched him on A and B. And, as many of you know, he has had a hard time finding his perfect match. Because his condition is deteriorating, he will most likely be transplanted with a donor who is not a perfect match. They will be a six of six but may not match on other, finer criteria. And, because time is short, he will not attempt to test those 800 four of four matches to see if the needle is really in the haystack.

Brian is not alone in facing this. About 95% of matches made through the NMDP are made with donors who were already typed at DR before the search began. That means that there are literally over a million donors who may never be called simply because to test them would take too long and cost too much, even though they might be better matches than the donors who are chosen.

We think no one should have to face the choice between a not-quite-perfect match and facing the time, health deterioration and expense of testing four of fours. If all of the donors in the registry were already typed at DR, then patients would have a head start finding the needle — that perfect-in-every-way donor. And while we can't fund DR typing for every donor in the registry, we can make a start. We hope that you will help us.

Date: Tue, 30 Mar 1999
**Subject: I like banging my head against the wall. It feels so good when
  you stop.**

We had sincerely hoped that this would be the update that gave you definite, firm info on when we are leaving for Brian's transplant. After all, this scheduling has been three weeks away for the last three months. "What could possibly go wrong this time?" we thought. Ha.

First, the molecular testing of the three remaining donors, which the lab swore would be done by yesterday, wasn't. And isn't. But that's OK, because they feel sufficiently certain of who his donor is going to be that, if Brian's doctor here would call and tell them his current clinical status, they would go ahead and schedule. No problem. Except that his doctor is on vacation until Tuesday. And the doctor who is covering for her is, understandably, unwilling to step in and start this process with someone else's patient unless it's a major emergency, which it's not. And we have been totally unable to convince the scheduling person to put him on the schedule without a call from his doctor, period, end of story.

So we're sitting here, Brian's platelets down to transfusion level once again, knowing that if either the testing was done or the doctors would talk to each other we could schedule, but unable to make that happen. What amazes me the most, I think, is that the folks at the transplant center don't seem to believe me when I tell them Brian's platelet count. One of them actually said to me, "If it were that low, his doctor would have called." Why would I make this up???????
AAAAAAAAAAAAAAAARGH! I have just spent about ten minutes taking out my aggressions on a pillow and the sofa in the back bedroom and feel somewhat better, but this is so FRUSTRATING! Why doesn't anything ever work the way it's supposed to in this stupid freaking situation?!?
So, we're in limbo again until next Tuesday, at least.

We are off to Boston tomorrow for Passover, where Eve will spend her first Seder with a sitter in her grandparents' bedroom because her cousins all either have or have been exposed to chicken pox, and we can't risk her getting them with Brian's transplant coming up. I know this is just the beginning, but when do we get our lives back?

OK, this concludes the update for those of you who don't live in Pittsburgh. If you live in the area, please read on.

We need your help. We are anticipating having to do a mountain of stuff when we get back from Boston in preparation for our departure. We desperately need volunteers who can spare an hour or two at a time to come over and play with Eve while we pack, make phone calls, do primal scream, or take a ten-minute walk to unwind. We simply need time on the calendar when we

24

know that someone else will be able to help with Eve. We don't need massive babysitting, just mother/father's helper sorts of things.

So, if you know of an afternoon or evening when you might be willing to come over and lend a hand for an hour, please e-mail me or call us and let us know. It will be greatly appreciated.

Thanks much for your help. Eve thanks you for any time you can spend tickling her tummy.

naomi

Ladies and gentleman, the moment you've all been waiting for . . .

We have a donor and a date! Finally! Oy!

Brian's donor is a 28 year-old Australian man, same blood type, CMV negative, and completely, fully, and utterly matched — the proverbial needle in a haystack.

Brian will have his first appointment on April 29th. He will begin his chemotherapy outpatient on May 13th or 14th, be admitted on the 17th or 18th, and have his transplant the 20th or 21st. In BMT jargon, one refers to days prior to transplant with negative numbers, transplant is day 0, and days post-transplant are positive numbers. So today is, roughly, day -42.

We will leave Pittsburgh sometime on the 26th. We are running around like maniacs trying to figure out how to pack everything up here, set everything up there and keep Eve from eating extension cords and dirt at the same time. What fun. Two days this week friends have come over to play with Eve while we get stuff done, which has been enormously helpful.

Thank you again for all your help and support.

naomi

Date: Mon, 19 Apr 1999
Subject: On your mark, get set . . .

So, here's the news from here:

We have been madly dashing around for the last ten days, scrambling to get things ready and get things set up in our apartment near the transplant center. We have had a steady stream of people taking care of Eve in the evenings, to the point where we actually have turned people away. We are profoundly grateful to all who have assisted. It may not feel like you're doing much, but you really are!

Thus far, we have booked our flights, arranged for transportation before we hook up with our car, rented an apartment, arranged for phone service, rented furniture and housewares, and mooched off of a friend for a crib and rocking chair for Eve.

We also put in a request today for Volunteer Services to hook us up with a volunteer family. The center has an amazing network of volunteers who are specially trained to be sensitive to the needs of BMT patients and families, and who act as "host families" for out-of-towners, taking them on outings and helping them with errands and whatnot. They ask you about a zillion questions about your interests and background when you sign up, and hopefully we'll make a nice contact in the area this way.

Brian's parents are here at the moment getting ready to drive our car out for us. They have rented a place in the same complex as us, and one or both of them will be there the whole time we are.

Brian, the spatial relations god, is busily packing the trunk of our car as we speak, making sure every last corner and crevice is filled. We are sending our computers out in the car, so I'm typing this from a loaned laptop because, as you all know, we develop tics if separated from e-mail for an extended period.

Brian has spent a great deal of time over the last couple of weeks putting together letters and videotapes for Eve. It may sound morbid, but he's given a lot of thought to the possibility that she may not remember him, and that he may not be around to influence her as she grows up. After much contemplation, he decided there were some specific things he wanted to say to her, and that if he didn't make it through transplant he still wanted to make sure they were said. So he's videotaped himself telling her some important stuff about his life, and he's written her a number of letters to be opened at specific points as she grows up. He hasn't let me in on what the tape or the letters say, but I think it's very touching that he wants to do it at all. He's a sensitive kind of guy, that husband of mine.

Now excuse me while I go wipe my eyes. I'm getting more than a little misty.

So, one week from today, we're off. And we have a request of all of you, which may sound a little weird.

Don't forget about us.

Oh, I know what you're thinking. "Don't be silly! You are on our minds!" I know. But we're going to be gone a long time, and while e-mails and calls and letters may come flowing in at the beginning, it's hard to keep that up. Frankly, we're both a little terrified that we're going to be doing this alone. We need to know you're with us. Brian has asked that a schedule be set up so he knows with certainty that he will get a call every day. Someone may soon be calling you to ask you to "subscribe." Please give generously.

Meanwhile, you can always reply to these e-mails. Keep in touch. A number of people have inquired about visiting. It's hard to know when a "good" time would be, because it is going to depend a lot on how Brian's doing. Whenever you come, we'll put you to work in the Brian and Eve caregiving rotation. Arduous tasks may also include taking me out to lunch. I know, it's rough.

Please be aware that if you have any kind of disease or infection, even a little sniffle, you will not be allowed into the BMT unit in the hospital, period, no exceptions, and won't be allowed to visit with Brian even out of the hospital. This is not a time to fudge it. You know if you are sick, and it is literally a life and death issue for Brian.

Oh, and while we're on the topic, Brian will not be able to accept fresh or dried flowers. Balloons and silk flowers are OK.

Well, that's what's going on here. Today I went for a massage, a gift from my mom, and my massage therapist had this to say about my stress level:
"You know, Naomi, most people's shoulder blades can move."

naomi

Date: Sat, 24 Apr 1999
Subject: Day -27: I love baldheaded men!

Well, only two more days until lift off. All of a sudden there has been an absolute outpouring of support for us, and it really has made a big difference. On Thursday, friends dropped by with matching Warner Brothers hats for us. Mine has Tweety Bird and the caption "Small Bird, Big Attitude" which seemed curiously appropriate. Eve has a pink Tweety hat with matching sunglasses. It is absurdly adorable. Brian's is for hospital wear. It says, "What's up, Doc?" Get it? I didn't. Duh.

Our friend, Nancy, has been coordinating a small number of Brian's friends to make sure he gets one phone call every day while we're away. She called yesterday to say, "Hey, what about you?" So she's now coordinating a similar effort on my behalf.

This morning at Shabbat morning services our Rabbi asked everyone to keep Brian, Eve and myself in mind as they sang the Mi Shebeirach — the prayer for healing. We weren't there because we have just a few things to do, but then, it wasn't us who was supposed to hear the prayer.

Also this morning, Nancy dropped by with a quilt she had made for us with beautiful quotations and prayers about friends stitched into it.

Then, this afternoon, well over thirty people came over to eat tons of sweets and watch Brian get his head shaved. Brian doesn't want anyone to say he looks terrible when his hair falls out, so he decided to speed the process along. We held a charity auction for the rights to have first crack at his hair to benefit Brian's fund at the HLA Registry. Michelle was our auctioneer, and it was an absolute riot. Her fine auctioneering skills were augmented by the fact that our Rabbi kept offering to up the bid if Michelle would do the shaving, which she wasn't willing to do. In the end, the final bid was $36 (which, in Judaism, is called a "double chai," meaning "double life"), with other people making dona-tions to bring the total money raised to $81. We also got a pledge of another $150.

Then the shaving began, and people took turns on poor Brian's head, making all kinds of wacky designs — the monk look, the reverse mohawk, striped beard, etc. I got to finish him off. He buzzed it all the way down but did-n't actually shave — not yet. He left a goatee and put on a clip-on hoop earring someone had sent. He bears a striking resemblance to Andre Agassi.

After the deed was done, Michelle borrowed my guitar and sang us a song she had written about our leaving — beautiful, and not a dry eye in the house.

We said many of our good-byes today, with more planned for tomorrow and Monday. This is becoming very real, but I think we are feeling more and more strengthened by the sheer volume of support. It also helps to remember that, even in this seemingly dark time, there's still some room to laugh and eat tiramisu. I'm not sure I could survive if there weren't.

Of course, this will ruin my whining that I have no friends and nobody loves me for some time to come, but I'll deal.

Thanks to one and all for all you've done. We will certainly be in touch, don't you worry!

naomi

Chapter 2:
The First 10 Million Appointments are the Hardest

Date: Wed, 28 Apr 1999
Subject: Day -23: I can't think of a cute subject line

Sunday was spent madly packing and arguing over whether one last sweatshirt would actually fit in our bags. Friends were over helping with Eve and sealing boxes, and they were unfortunately privy to some very ugly scenes, which they seemed to find very amusing. Brian and I are still married, you'll be happy to know, although it was touch and go for a while there.

At one o'clock on Monday, the caravan to the airport began. It took two cars to get us and all our junk to the airport — six suitcases, stroller, booster seat, car seat, a box, a knapsack, camcorder, oy. And that doesn't even start to address all the stuff we shipped.

Our flight was not nonstop — we had a connection in Philadelphia. Before you all go scrambling for your maps, I can affirm that Philadelphia is exactly in the wrong direction. However, when you're flying on free frequent flyer tickets, you take what they give you. All of us had one stage of a cold or another, and take-offs and landings were especially hard on Eve's ears. She cried all the way down on both legs of the flight.

By the time we finally got in it was 8:45 PM local time, 11:45 our time, we were exhausted, and Eve had completely had it. I couldn't blame her for crying because I was getting pretty fussy myself.

We were met at the airport by Heather and Randal, our volunteer family. Heather and Randal are a youngish (our age, so you can call that young or not depending on your point of view) engaged couple who seem, well, pretty much like us. They helped us get our luggage (which, oddly, appeared to have arrived on an earlier flight, although we can't for the life of us figure out how) and drove us to our apartment, where Brian's parents were already waiting for us, having arrived a day earlier with our car.

The furniture and housewares were already here, and Barb and Joe (Brian's parents) had bought us a few things to get us through the first night. They had even put flowers on the table. All we had to do was make the bed and go to sleep. The latter was not hard. Because we had sent our own linens with Barb and Joe, we had the pleasure of snuggling into bed under our own sheets and a quilt my sister-in-law made for us for our wedding. I was also reunited with Ollie, my stuffed hippo who travels everywhere with me (he was even present at Eve's birth, I have witnesses). All of this added up to making us feel just a little more at home than expected, which was nice.

Our apartment is a two-bedroom on the corner of the 13th floor, four blocks from the outpatient clinic. We have a relatively nice view and can even see a little piece of water. At night, the lights of the city are quite beautiful. We get a lot of sun, especially in the afternoon, which keeps the place very warm. The apartment isn't huge, but it's quite adequate and we don't feel like we're camping out. We can actually live here.

Yesterday, we spent the day getting things connected and set up and doing grocery shopping. We met our friend Mark for lunch. Mark is a close friend who is a former student in Brian's department. He works within walking distance of our apartment. He also came over for dinner last night. Can you tell we're glad to see each other?

Today was more shopping — buy stock in Target — and I rented a breast pump so I can provide milk for Eve on the many occasions I'll be off taking care of Brian and can't be there to nurse her.

The major problem of our lives right now is the fact that we don't have a parking space for the car. There's a one-month waiting list for the parking lot associated with our building, and the lot down the street where we had planned to park it is no longer accepting monthly leases. However, Heather (of Heather and Randal, above) is working on finding someplace for us.

We've had a few calls from friends at home and family, which has been a treat. It's hard to remember that just because we aren't where we usually are doesn't mean the phone doesn't work, but every time it rings it's a little surprise.

Well, this has been way longer than I had intended, so I guess I had better finish it up. We'll be back to medical stuff with tomorrow's update.

naomi

I awoke this morning with a cough and a runny nose — second cold of the week and a definitive killer for our dinner plans. We had planned on going to the home of another "transplant couple" to have dinner with them and some other patients we had also met on the Internet. However, since my cold is in the "extremely yucky" stage (a medical term), we thought it was best not to risk giving it to others.

This afternoon, we left Eve with Barb and Joe and proceeded up to the clinic for Brian's first appointment. Since both of us have colds, we are really unwelcome in the clinic and had to sit outside the main waiting room while Brian filled out his forms. They then took us in a "back way" (actually, we've never been in the front way, since Brian had a cold the last time we were here, too) for Brian's appointment with the current Fellow on the Red Team.

There are around eight teams here, and you are assigned to one when you start your transplant process based on the type of transplant you are having. All of the teams have color names, although Red seems to be one of the more boring ones. Others have names like Aqua or Violet. We agreed we'd much rather be on the Burnt Sienna team, or, perhaps, the Banana team.

Anyway, the Fellow took Brian's history, which Brian is thinking of committing to an audio tape so he doesn't actually have to be at these appointments, and listened to his chest, etc. We then met with one of the Red Team nurses, who came in wearing a gown and mask because, due to his cold, Brian is now in "isolation," meaning that he must now be treated as though he has the plague until his nose stops dripping. She drew approximately 17 trillion vials of blood and then cultured his sinuses to make sure that this really is a cold and not the aforementioned plague. Culturing his sinuses consisted of putting saline up his nose and then having him snort into a cup. If you think that's gross, consider that they used to do this manually using a cotton swab.

The nurse gave us a big manual of everything we could ever hope to know about the transplant program, lots and lots of consent forms to read over before tomorrow's big pow-wow with the attending physician, and the schedule of Brian's tests and appointments for tomorrow and most of next week.

On our way out of the clinic, a total stranger came over and addressed me by name. This may not seem like a big deal to those of you named Bob or Mary, but there aren't too many Naomis in the world, so this was a rather unnerving experience. Turns out it was Jack Sarfaty, a fellow member of my BMT Internet mailing list and one of the people we had originally planned to have dinner with tonight. He had seen Brian's name on a folder and put two and two together. It was nice to put a face with a name, and, since his transplant is scheduled for only a week or so before Brian's, I'm sure we'll be seeing him a lot.

Brian then went off for a chest X-ray while I came home to rescue Barb and Joe from Little Miss Separation Anxiety. Alternately, I went home so they could rescue Brian from Big Mrs. Separation Anxiety. Depends upon your point of view.

No sooner had Brian returned from his X-ray when the clinic called to say his platelet count was down and he needed to come back this evening for a transfusion. The four of us killed some time and then he and Barb went back to the clinic. He called after an hour to say that the blood bank had sent over the wrong platelets so he was going to be a while. This gave us a sense of familiarity. It seems the same screw-ups happen no matter where you are!

Meanwhile, back at the ranch, the church across the street has given us preliminary permission to park in their lot, and Randal and Heather, our volunteers, managed to find most of the child-proofing stuff we hadn't been able to get our paws on yet. So at least some things are working out. It's very nice to have someone assigned to solve the stupid problems we don't have time to deal with. It's not that we couldn't do these things, but it's wonderful not to have to.

Having a volunteer family is also a little weird because I'm the sort of person who tends to volunteer for these kinds of organizations. It's strange to be on the receiving end rather than the giving end of the help. There's part of me that feels we don't deserve it. Our finances are OK, and Brian isn't in the hospital yet. On the other hand, just having someone assigned to care about you takes a lot of the emotional burden away. I wonder if these volunteers know how much of a difference they make just by doing the small stuff.

It's been so nice to hear from a few of you via phone, mail and e-mail. Thanks for keeping in touch. It really does help to know that someone is actually out there reading this stuff.

More tomorrow. . . .

naomi

34

Date: Fri, 30 Apr 1999
Subject: Day -21

Another day, another 10 million appointments.

This morning, Brian, accompanied by Joe, went up to the ambulatory clinic to meet with the nutritionist and have a pulmonary function test. The nutritionist was apparently quite impressed with Brian. He drinks lots of juice and milk, he eats several small meals a day and he doesn't take weird supplements that interfere with medication. The nutritionist also felt that his exercise level was good. Yes, he really does do *Tae Bo*, although I solemnly swear I did not buy it from the infomercial.

Brian was pleased to learn that the inpatient wards offer 24 hour "room service," and the attitude of the nutritionist was, essentially, "If you want to eat, who are we to stop you?" Most BMT patients have horrendous problems with nausea and appetite. Brian shared with her my experience eating Cap'n Crunch Berries during my pregnancy because it was the only thing that would go down. She said that there are many similarities between coping with transplant nausea and coping with severe morning sickness. It's nice to know I have skills that may become useful.

Brian then proceeded to his pulmonary function test, where it was determined that his pulmonaries are functioning, or something. He blew into various tubes while they did various things to him, and his lungs seem to be in good shape, which was not a surprise.

Meanwhile, Eve and I went and made some copies and opened a bank account specifically for the money that is still in dispute which we have received from the insurance company. I will spare the gory details, but suffice it to say that our battle about coverage for Brian's search is not over. It may never be. Hundreds of years from now, there will be a distant Zikmund-Fisher great great great grandchild still trying to settle our estate. Our insurer will still be refusing to let him or her talk to anyone except the folks in Customer Service who won't even give out their last name, let alone a direct phone number.

In the afternoon, we went up to the clinic for Brian's arrival conference. We met for an hour or so with the attending physician on the Red Team. This was nice, although all of the doctors will be rotating in the next week so we'll get to meet a whole new set. We talked some about the plan for Brian's treatment, some clinical studies they would like him to participate in, and what he can expect in the next few weeks. It seemed like this conference was pretty much set up for patients and caregivers who aren't really sure they want to have a transplant, so we learned relatively little that was new to us. It was a little unnerving to discover that, after one consult six months ago and one intake appointment yesterday, we already have a reputation for knowing a lot. I wish I had the confidence in us that they all seem to have.

35

Brian then went for a blood draw before our last date of the day with Melody, our patient finance guru. This meeting was mostly spent swapping stories about how awful our insurance company is and her conveying her hope that they would be less of a pain about what lies ahead than they were about his search coverage. Our insurer has, miracle of miracles, already pre-approved the transplant, so we don't anticipate much of a problem. Unlike some people with less insurance or less cooperative (if you can imagine such a thing) insurance, we don't have to put up a huge deposit before the transplant.

I was talking to a friend earlier this week and she expressed concern that Brian's transplant wouldn't be covered. She was afraid that, since we changed insurance plans in November, they wouldn't cover a pre-existing condition. Now, there are a bunch of legal reasons why they can't do that, not to mention that my union contract specifically states that our insurance has to cover pre-existing conditions. But that isn't the point. The point is, do people really think we're dumb enough that we wouldn't have checked that out? I mean, I know things don't always go as planned, but don't you think we would probably have at least tried to look into this? Grumble, grumble, grumble.

Moving along, in the late afternoon, Barb, Joe, Brian, Eve and I went across the street to the church, which maintains a "lending closet" for transplant families. When I heard about this, I imagined a small, dingy closet with a few broken down, non-functional items which one would only use if desperate. Boy, was I wrong! The "closet" is a large storage room with tons of housewares, furniture, bedding, baby items, etc. Our first reaction upon walking in was, "Why did we rent stuff at all?" We certainly could have outfitted our kitchen completely from the closet. As it was, we left with several useful items such as fans, a laundry basket, and Tupperware.

On another note, the four year-old daughter of some friends explained to a playmate that Uncle Brian has to take medicine that might make his hair fall out, so instead of taking the medicine, he shaved his head. She also explained that right now he has green and blue blood cells, and he has to go to the hospital to get red and white ones. Which is actually, if you think about it, not such a bad explanation!

naomi

Date: Mon, 3 May 1999
Subject: Day -18

Brian had no clinic appointments this weekend, so we took the opportunity to eat our way across the city and otherwise kick back a little. Friday night we found a little Ethiopian place. We figure communal plate restaurant food is pretty much the epitome of what Brian will not be allowed to eat pretty soon.

Saturday morning, Cliff, Carol, Luke and Megan Slaughterbeck came over. Carol had an autologous (i.e. she got her own cells rather than cells from a donor) stem cell transplant for breast cancer in December, and I met Cliff through BMT-talk, an Internet mailing list. We met Cliff and Carol in person in November when we were out for Brian's consult. The Slaughterbecks and various of their coworkers and friends are lending us baby furniture for Eve, and they dropped it off and stayed for a visit while Cliff and Brian did the "guy thing" and assembled everything.

Yesterday, Heather and Randal took us for a driving tour around the city.

Last night, we celebrated my birthday nine days early with a "date" (read, "no Eve") at the best steak house in town. Brian wanted to get a really good rare steak, since rare meat will be off the menu probably for several months to a year.

This morning it was back to reality. Brian had an 8 AM (ugh) appointment to begin his work-up. The purpose of the work-up is to get a baseline reading on all parts of Brian's health before transplant so they can do comparisons after transplant. They also want to make sure that there aren't any heretofore-undiscovered medical issues that might make him a poor candidate for transplant.

Because my cold, although much better, has developed into a hacking cough, I got to wear a fetching yellow mask throughout this appointment. Brian had a bone marrow biopsy, a blood draw, in which they took about ten zillion tubes of blood, and an EKG. They also took rectal and nasal swabs to culture to see what bugs he carries around normally which might pose a problem when his immune system is suppressed.

This was Brian's 6th bone marrow biopsy (BMB) and by far the easiest. At home, when he has a BMB, they give him Ativan®, which is an anti-anxiety medication. This helps him feel relaxed during the procedure, but it's still really painful. Today, they gave him fentanyl, a fast-acting narcotic. They injected it, and within 10 seconds he was in a happy place. They did the biopsy, but from the look on his face I would have thought they had only just begun when they were done. Brian said this was the first time he would describe what he experienced as "discomfort" instead of "excruciating indescribable pain."

The immediate loopiness from the drug wore off within about 15 minutes, and we came back to the apartment, although he did nap for awhile. Brian is now a major devotee of this drug. Frankly, I am too. It's much easier to

37

watch the biopsy being done when you think of the nurse as having gotten your sweetie stoned rather than as trying to kill your sweetie.

Brian's EKG came out as "borderline," so it will be looked at by a cardiologist. The nurse said that a huge number of them come out as "borderline" and almost none of them actually have a problem. She said we could rest assured that Brian does, indeed, have a heart and that it is the correct size, unlike the Grinch's. (You know, the Grinch's heart was two sizes too small. She really said that, I'm not making this up!)

At the end of the appointment, I discovered, much to my embarrassment, that I had the stupid mask on upside down. So much for being suave and sophisticated. I think I'm losing it.

Thanks to all for listening and keeping in touch. Please know that when you call and write, even if we can't talk to you right then, it really makes a difference in how we feel about this whole experience. OK, I know I keep saying that. I'm trying to provide positive reinforcement for successive approximations of the desired behavior. I need you. The thread I'm hanging by may get thicker and thinner, but it's still a thread.

naomi

Some of you have asked me to present a brief overview of Brian's current situation, his treatment plan and what lies ahead in terms of risks and complications.

So, let's begin from the beginning.

Brian has myelodysplastic syndrome, or MDS. This is a progressive, life-threatening bone marrow disorder in which the marrow does not properly differentiate the various types of blood cells, meaning he doesn't have enough of any of them. This is bad.
MDS can and often does proceed to AML, a form of leukemia. However, Brian has shown no signs of this progression. This is good.
At the moment, Brian is being kept alive by receiving platelet transfusions. Without these, he runs a risk of spontaneous and uncontrollable bleeding, which would, I think you'd agree, be bad. But one cannot receive transfusions forever. After a while the body stops accepting the foreign cells.

The only potential long-term cure for MDS is a bone marrow transplant to kill off the diseased marrow and replace it with healthy stuff.
In order to do this, he will receive extremely high doses of chemotherapy, which will attack all of his cells but in particular rapidly dividing ones, which includes those in his marrow. He will then receive bone marrow from his donor. The donor will not travel here. He will have his surgery in Australia on either an outpatient or a one-night-stay basis, and the marrow will be flown here by courier. We will have no direct contact with the donor for at least one year, although we can send letters and updates without identifying information.
The transplant is not a surgical procedure. The marrow cells actually "know" where to go, so they are transfused like a blood transfusion and, we hope, begin to grow when they hit the marrow space. The donor will have surgery, but Brian won't.

The relapse rate for Brian's type of MDS is very low — maybe 1 or 2%. If this works, it should really work. Even transplants that are flawless, however, have a lot of nasty side effects. The most common ones worth mentioning are hair loss (everybody loses their hair, period), and mucositis, or sores on the mucous membranes of the mouth and digestive tract. It is anticipated that Brian will stop being able to eat and drink due to mucositis, at which time he will receive total parenteral nutrition (TPN), an IV form of nutrition.

There are other complications that range from annoying to life threatening, and I will attempt to run them down:

Infection — Between the time when Brian's marrow is destroyed and the new stuff is working, he will have no immune system at all, so any infection is a life threatening infection. He will get tons of antibiotics, antifungals, antivirals, etc. to fight infections and will be cultured up the wazoo (what part of the body is the wazoo?) to catch things before they become a problem. Even after his new marrow starts to engraft, infection will still be a big risk.

Graft-versus-Host Disease (GVHD) — The vast majority of unrelated donor transplant patients have some form of GVHD. In this disease, the new immune system looks around and says, "Hey, there's all sorts of stuff around here that's foreign. Let's kill it." The problem is, all that stuff is the patient. GVHD can range from mild to life threatening. Brian will take immunosuppressive drugs to fight it, but those increase the risk of infection. It's a balancing act. He will probably be on these drugs for at least a year, and possibly much more. During this entire time, Brian will have restrictions on his diet and on certain types of public activities to reduce his exposure to germs.

Graft Failure — This is the opposite, in some ways, of GVHD. The patient's body looks at the donor's marrow and says, "That's not mine," and the new marrow does not grow. This is fairly uncommon, especially when the match between donor and patient is good, but it is pretty much the worst thing that can happen.

Veno-Occlusive Disease — This is a complication of the liver, which generally occurs in the first month after transplant and is potentially life threatening.

As you can see, there is a lot to look for and a lot of meds to take. Brian will be in the hospital beginning a couple of days before transplant until his absolute neutrophil count (ANC), a measure of mature white cells, is up out of the danger level and until his nausea and mucositis have subsided to the point where he can take some nutrition by mouth. He will then be back at the apartment and monitored closely as an outpatient for two or so months.

Through this all, Brian will have a Hickman catheter, which is essentially a permanent IV which he will have placed in his chest so he doesn't have to keep getting poked. After he's out of the hospital, he will still be receiving meds, nutrition, and hydration through this central line, so we will learn how to use pumps and care for the Hickman at home.

Brian can expect to be "out of commission" to a greater or lesser extent for a year or even more. Everyone's different, of course, but this is a long road.

Anyway, I hope this answered some of the bigger questions. I'm happy to answer any others you may have.

naomi

40

Brian's day began this morning with an exciting visit to Oral Medicine. It is really important that Brian's teeth and mouth be in good shape before transplant so he doesn't begin the process with any latent infections or weird germs. They took a full set of x-rays on the cool machine that goes around and around your head, and then the Resident, followed by the attending, poked at his mouth.

The senior doctors are called "attending" physicians. They supervise "Resident" physicians who have graduated medical school and are licensed, but are completing their specialized training. There are also a lot of "Fellows" around here, who have done their Residency, usually in Internal Medicine, and are now doing even more training. The Residents and Fellows get most of the grudge work, while the attendings get to review the grudge work and redo it as necessary.

Anyway, while all this examining was going on, I filled out a form about Brian's dental habits. Brian was very annoyed that I didn't ask him for the answers, but let's face it, I know how often he goes to the dentist and I buy his mouthwash myself. The first thing they told him was to stop using alcohol-based mouthwash. Apparently, the alcohol in most mouthwashes is not good for mucositis because it dries the mucosa (the things that get inflamed during mucositis), so they want him off it well before transplant.

They then started taking a look at his mouth, and, in particular, at a sore on his lip which appeared in the last few days. It wasn't at all clear what it was, so the attending ordered a culture of it to see if it's yeast, a cold sore, some sort of bacterial infection or what, so they can treat it appropriately. If a healthy person got this type of sore, they would use some extra Blistex® and not really think about it, but for someone in Brian's situation every little thing has to be reported and treated.

Pending results of the culture, they prescribed an anti-bacterial rinse for Brian to use in place of his mouthwash and scheduled him to come back tomorrow to talk more about the sore. Otherwise his teeth look fine.

We then went to an exam room where Brian had another "Isolation Blood Draw" since we haven't managed to shake our colds quite yet. We keep thinking one more day, but it hasn't happened yet. Believe it or not, they managed to forget two tubes they needed yesterday, so he had to have more blood drawn today, making a total of something like 17 tubes in the last two days. I suppose that is only going to get worse, but it's pretty impressive.

We then had a lengthy appointment with our Social Worker, Moreen. Her job is to be our advocate and help us through the maze of stuff here and also to help us through the emotional side of things. She interviewed us extensively about our backgrounds, relationship, coping mechanisms, support systems, styles of dealing with doctors, families, etc. This was really a very helpful meeting for both of us, because it gave us a chance to sort of examine how we are doing emotionally and what we need more help with. After some discussion, we decided that, although she is always available if we need to talk, we are really unlikely to admit we need to talk, so she's arranging for us to be scheduled to see her individually on a regular basis. She is also arranging for Pastoral Care to have a local Rabbi get in touch with us.

In the afternoon, we had planned for Barb and Joe to go take the first of a series of caregiving classes or, if their colds weren't gone, for us to go. However, our colds aren't gone either and we can't be around other patients, so we will have to take this class next week.

Best to all, and tune in tomorrow!

naomi

Date: Wed, 5 May 1999
Subject: Day -16

Brian woke up this morning saying, "I don't feel too good." He was coughing up a storm and his nose was very stuffed — definitely a turn for the worse. I, on the other hand, seemed to be in the very last stages of this cold. We called the Red Team scheduler and told her we were a no go for today's transplant classes, and she cancelled us out of tomorrow's as well. We'll try again next week. I know that's not a big deal, but I actually felt rejected when she said she was going to cancel our classes. I felt like she somehow thought it was our fault we continued to be sick. I really am losing it.

We also spoke to the Red Team RN and she said she thought the doctors ought to take another peek at Brian and see what was going on in his sinuses. We went up to the clinic right after lunch, following our usual isolation routine. The schedule called for 12:30 meeting with Pain and Toxicity, 1:00 follow-up with Oral Medicine, a quick blood draw and now for the Red Team docs to take a look at Brian.

We arrived at 12:30 and sat. After 20 minutes I went back out to reception, and they paged Pain and Tox again. Finally, at 12:55 the doctor came in and talked for about half an hour with Brian about his prior experiences with chemo and radiation (none), prior drug or alcohol abuse (none), prior problems with anesthesia (none), etc. Pain and Tox are the doctors responsible for pain relief, nausea relief, anesthesia and the like. They will be helping Brian with these problems as he proceeds through transplant, and they want to get to know him ahead of time.

As P and T was finishing up (it was now 1:25 or so), Dr. M., the new Red Team Fellow, came in and talked to Brian about his cold. He listened to Brian's lungs, told us the sinus culture from Thursday hadn't turned up anything nasty and said he thought Brian should go for another chest X-ray and possibly a sinus CT. He left, saying he'd be back in "a second." It was now 1:45.

At around 2:05, I went out to reception and pointed out that a) Dr. M. seemed to have been abducted, b) Brian still needed his isolation blood draw and c) the Oral Medicine people probably thought Brian had been abducted. Chuck, the much beloved receptionist, paged everyone in creation, and I went back to the room. The lab came and drew blood, and we sat.

At 2:25, I went back out to Chuck, who again paged around.

At 2:40, I was on my way out to the bathroom when I ran into the Red Team RN. She was able to find out in about 30 seconds that Dr. M. wanted Brian to go over for a Chest X-ray and got him the orders to allow that to happen. She didn't know why no one had told him that or why Dr. M. had never come back. Shortly thereafter, Oral Medicine came by to say that the cultures

43

on Brian's mouth sore weren't back anyway, so it was just as well that he missed his appointment. The clerk form Oral Medicine said she'd be "right back" with a time for a rescheduled appointment tomorrow.

I bet you know where this is going. . . .

After 15 minutes, when she hadn't returned, we left. I told Chuck in a rather, um, animated manner, that they could leave the info on our answering machine, which they didn't — we had to call back. Very aggravating. I left a message for Moreen expressing some con-CERN about being left to fester in an examining room all afternoon.

Brian had his chest X-ray, and we decided to take advantage of a gorgeous afternoon to go to the park. Eve absolutely loved this. She especially liked it when Daddy pushed her on the swings — the giggling got a lot of attention from passers by. It was a nice break from apartment confinement and there was a lot for her to see. She took this opportunity to stand alone for lengthy periods of time, and even took two consecutive steps. She did such a convincing impression of a baby who walks, she almost had everyone fooled. After this abortive walking attempt, she kept standing up and falling down flat on her face — she just can't quite do it yet.

When we returned, there was a message on our machine saying that Brian's donor got the official and final clearance to donate today, so, provided Brian's cold goes away in finite time, he should be a go for starting chemo on the 14th and transplant on the 21st.

I also received e-mail today from the HLA Registry telling me that Brian's fund has now raised over $1600 for DR typing. That's enough to DR type about 50 donors. We are really pleased with how this is going so far, and yet there is always more to do! Thanks to all who have contributed. You are amazing.

Tonight we had Mark over for dinner and then went to an ice cream place recommended by our volunteer family. Heather and Randal are obviously a very good family for us. Anyone who can recommend good ice cream is OK by me. All in all, it was a nice ending to a really annoying day.

naomi

Yesterday was a light schedule. Brian had an appointment with the Oral Medicine department to go over the results of the cultures on his mouth sore. I stayed home to commune with Eve. We've pretty much been attached at the hip since she was born, and it's hard to leave her virtually every day, even if only for a couple of hours. We had a nice time just hanging out and pretending life is normal.

It's taken us a while to get into a groove as far as my in-laws babysitting goes. I admit that my father-in-law, in particular, is doing a much better job than I thought he would. The night of Brian's first platelet transfusion here I announced to Brian that under no circumstances was I leaving Eve alone with Joe. After all, he doesn't do things exactly and precisely the way I do. How shocking! Actually, Eve is quickly warming up to Joe and he seems to be really enjoying her, so this will be OK. But still, in-laws are in-laws and, frankly, they drive me a little crazy.

Brian arrived home from his Oral Medicine appointment to find me on the phone. I was somewhat absorbed, so Brian started playing with Eve. He stood her up in the hall, moved away, and said, "Walk to Daddy!" Well, she did. It was very dramatic — four whole steps. That's my girl!

We spent the rest of yesterday running errands and then continued on our quest to eat our way across the city. Brian picked Mongolian Barbecue. This is quite a change for the guy who thinks we eat out too much, but he figures that if we average this week with the next six months, we're still eating out less than we were before.

This morning we went up to the clinic for a blood draw (how unusual) and a "clinic appointment." Clinic appointments are basically just a routine visit with the doctors. Since the doctors just rotated, this was our chance to meet the new guys. We had met the Fellow during that infamous "let's sit in the exam room forever" incident on Wednesday, but not the attending.

This appointment was pretty much uneventful, since he hasn't actually had any treatment yet. They talked to Brian about his cold. It is getting better and seems to have been helped by the antibiotics he's been taking in preparation for his transplant, which suggests he had a little sinus infection or something. They looked at the various red bumps that have appeared on his head and decreed them to be folliculitis — irritated hair follicles caused by his recent shaving exploits. There's a problem he won't have in a few weeks. They also gave us the preliminary reports of his last marrow, which still show no blasts — great news.

Dr. M. was extremely apologetic about leaving us stranded in the exam room for more than an hour on Wednesday. I would even say he was graceful about it. Moreen had clearly said something to him about it. He admitted that he had, indeed, been abducted by aliens and probed, but he was feeling much better other than the little thing sticking out of the back of his neck (I'm not making this up, he really said this).

We also got a chance to meet the new Red Team attending. We traded stories about "hot tub folliculitis," an irritation of the hair follicle caused by bacteria in hot tubs which Brian and I both had just before our wedding. She said that now she will remember Brian well — the folliculitis guy.

This afternoon we went in search of Shabbat candles. In Judaism, Shabbat (the Sabbath) begins on Friday night with the lighting of candles to symbolize the fire the Israelites lit in their camp before the Sabbath so they wouldn't have to work at building a fire during their day of rest. There's a standard sized candle which is used for this, but we haven't been able to find them out here. In fact, we didn't manage to find them again today. I need to ask the local Rabbi where to get them nearby.

We stopped by the outdoor market to buy some fish and I also bought Brian a necklace with the Viking runes for "Journey" and "Growth" (which symbolizes rebirth) to add to his burgeoning collection of neckwear. He's been wearing a necklace that a friend gave him that says "courage" and "wisdom" on it. These seemed like good additions.

When we came home I went off to give blood — and if you gave the last time I noodged, you're due too. I admit that I'm becoming a blood and marrow zealot. I am losing all sympathy for people who are eligible and who don't give blood and aren't marrow donors. During Brian's search, one friend wanted to get typed just for Brian, but refused to go into the registry. I just don't understand that. The stranger whose life you might save is just as precious to his friends and family as Brian is to us!

OK, sorry, I'm calm now.

We were just about to settle down to Shabbat dinner when the nurse from the clinic called to say that Brian's ANC, a measure of the mature white cells, was well into the danger zone for infection. This is the lowest ANC he's ever had. So they put him on a broad-spectrum antibiotic, to add to the collection of pill bottles on the counter, and he has to have blood draws both weekend days.

My response to the low ANC was almost Pavlovian — "Oh my God! ANC low! Run in circles, scream and shout!" My heart started beating faster and my stomach flipped. When I thought about it, however, I realized that the main reason this scared me hearkened back to the months after Eve was born. Brian's counts were fairly stable at that time and he decided to put off his transplant until they dipped. His doctor gave him thresholds for each of his counts at which she felt transplant would become necessary. Although his platelet count passed the "transplant necessary" point months ago, today was the first day his ANC dipped below its threshold. So my reaction was basically a knee-jerk, "Oh my God, he's going to need a transplant" reaction which, upon reflection, was

46

not news.

No hot plans for the weekend other than more eating and blood draws. Sunday is my first Mother's Day, and if I'm really good Brian won't let Eve cook me breakfast in bed.

naomi

Date: Mon, 10 May 1999
Subject: Day -11: Ergh!!

This weekend we had a little less "off time" than last weekend. Saturday morning, Brian went for a blood draw to check his platelets and neutrophils, and then we went with Mark on a lovely ferry ride. While on the ferry, Brian was paged by the clinic to say that his platelets were down and he needed to be transfused. He scheduled that for after dinner.

Meanwhile, his mother was out for a walk and that pesky sidewalk, totally unprovoked, jumped up and bit her on the face. So she became the first member of the family to see the hospital emergency room, beating Brian by a good measure. She had five stitches and is fine, although her pride has suffered some casualties. I don't think she imagined that, of the five of her family members out here, the one having trouble learning to walk would be her. First day on the new feet, I guess.

The people keeping an eye on our house in Pittsburgh called to say that the sewer was backing up in our basement, how lovely, so we had to try to get that taken care of at a 2500-mile distance. I suppose I should be really upset about this, but a) it's a rental and b) I'm not there smelling it. Call me cynical, I don't mind.

Saturday night, Brian had his last sushi dinner for a long, long time. Uncooked fish is not at the top of the "safe to eat if your immune system is compromised" list. He then had his Saturday night transfusion, which is not, I think it is safe to say, his favorite way to spend a Saturday night. I try to remind myself the whole reason for doing this transplant, strange as it seems, is so he won't have to spend any more Saturday nights, days, or any other day of the week getting transfused anymore. He came home and we all went to bed, a long day.

Yesterday was Mother's Day, a long time coming for me. Eve's conception was the result of a long and emotional struggle with infertility, and Mother's Day was always a very difficult day for me in the past. It seems amazing to finally be celebrating and incredible the circumstances under which I'm doing it. We thought our days of scouring the country for the best care for complex and emotionally draining medical problems was over the day I found out I was pregnant. Ha.

Brian went for a blood draw again Sunday morning, and then he and Joe and Eve took me and Barb out for lunch. Unfortunately, something in the buffet did not agree with either of us (or, alternately, we both have a little stomach bug). At any rate, I felt slightly yucky and Brian has had abdominal cramping for two days. Buffets are a big no-no when it comes to food safety for BMT patients, and I think we discovered why!

Of course, a little tummy upset is a nuisance for anyone, but for a transplant patient it's a big deal. So this morning, in addition to his regularly sched-

48

uled appointments, Brian had to get this checked. The good news is that, since his cold is over, he is out of isolation, and so he got to see the lower halves of the staff's faces at clinic today instead of just their masks.

I had an appointment with Moreen, the social worker, this morning, which seemed to alarm Chuck, the receptionist. He felt there must be some implications for our marriage that Brian and I are seeing her separately. Truth is, this affects us both in different ways.

What did we talk about? Everything and nothing. About being away from home. About the possibility that Brian might die. About trying to get along with Brian's parents. About the fact that I'm actually doing OK, which makes me think that something must be seriously wrong with me. Mostly, it was good to have some time that was just mine to talk. On the one hand, I know that it's Brian who's sick, and I don't want to make this whole thing about me when it's really about him. On the other hand, it's not like it doesn't affect me at all.

Meanwhile, the nurse checked his blood pressure and talked to him about his stomach. As Brian puts it, the clinic's view of all problems is, "Let's get a culture of that." This includes when you have the runs, which is not the most pleasant thing one could have to do, but he did. He refuses to share with me how he did it and, frankly, I don't really want him to draw me a picture.

While we were waiting for him to be seen by the doctor, I went over to see his scheduler. Before he can start chemo, Brian needs to have surgery to place his Hickman catheter, the central line in his chest through which he will receive blood, fluids, medications, nutrition and his new marrow, and out of which they can draw blood. He also needs to have a final review conference with the doctor to go over the results of all the tests they've done and sign consents. These two things hadn't appeared on our schedule, so I went to ask the scheduler why they hadn't been scheduled. She said they were waiting for "final confirmation of the date." I nearly came unglued. The date was confirmed last Wednesday as far as we knew, and if Brian can't get his chemo started on time they might have to put off his transplant. And if his donor can't donate the next day or the day after that, it could be weeks or even longer!

When Dr. M. (or the alien who took his place) came to see Brian, I expressed some, um, con-CERN about this. He told me not to worry about it. Three times. I told him he must not know me very well. Why would I ask if I wasn't worried already?

By the way, it turns out that when Dr. M. left us sitting in the exam room forever last week, he was working on a code. That's code, as in "code blue." In other words, he was resuscitating someone. So I think we forgive him. I also think the notion that someone coded while in the outpatient clinic is a little scarier than I like to contemplate. Aren't people in outpatient supposed to be the relatively healthy ones? Do you mean you can get out of the hospital and then just drop dead? I don't even want to think about it. So let's move on.

We went out to lunch with the Slaughterbecks after clinic. Carol was there for an experimental cancer vaccine they are giving her to try to prevent relapse of her breast cancer. We went to a deli that has what I consider soul food. For me, soul food is kosher corned beef, bagel and lox and matza brie. Everyone's different. Now at least I know where to get comfort food. I'm sure I'll need it.

After lunch, I called the nurse for Brian's team and left a message expressing, um, con-CERN about the schedule, and we headed out to the mall where Brian, for some unknown reason, seemed to need to do some shopping. You'd think someone's birthday was tomorrow or something. Not mentioning any names . . .

When we returned this afternoon, there was a message from the scheduler with the times for the conference and the Hickman placement. Of course these times conflict with our class schedule, so I'll be taking make-ups after Brian's in the hospital. Whatever. There was another message from the Red Team Nurse apologizing for the misunderstanding. I fear I am getting a reputation for my, um, con-CERN about things. Well, they'll have to live with it.

Sorry this is so long — sometimes you gotta ramble so you don't go completely nuts. Thanks for listening! More tomorrow.

naomi

Date: Tue, 11 May 1999
Subject: Day -10: Happy Birthday to Me

Today began with Brian and Eve, for some reason lost in 29 years worth of the sands of time, showering me with gifts.

In the afternoon, we went to the clinic for the first half of "Introduction to Managing Care," a basic class about going through transplant. We learned nothing new, but the class reinforced a few basics, such as 1) Wash your hands 2) No fresh flowers 3) Wash your hands 4) Brian can't change diapers 5) Wash your hands and 6) Wash your hands.

If you came to visit us right now, you might think we've become a tad compulsive. The rule is, everyone in our home must wash their hands with soap when they arrive, after using the bathroom, after coughing or sneezing into their hands, after wiping or blowing their nose, after touching their mouth, after doing any of the above with Eve, after changing her diaper, etc. Buy stock in cosmetic companies, because we are using a ton of lotion to prevent dry skin. All this hand washing may seem extreme, but research shows that this is the single most effective protection against the spread of infection.

We ducked out of class half way through to go to Brian's data review conference with the Red Team attending. She went over the results of all his many tests, and said, "Aside from a little MDS, you're in great shape!" Brian signed a slew of consent forms for various research studies. He'll be getting a newer treatment as part of a randomized trial of drugs to prevent fungal infections. He'll also be allowing them to take two extra teaspoons of his blood from time to time for a huge number of other studies. Most of these studies will not affect him really at all, but may help others like him in the future.

Tomorrow, Brian has his Hickman placed at 6 AM (ugh) and meets with the nurse to discuss how to take his busulfan, the first chemo drug which starts on Friday. Thursday he starts his Dilantin®, an anti-seizure medication he has to take with busulfan. Friday he reports at 7:45 AM and the games begin: four days of busulfan during which he has to be at clinic for almost 7 hours each day as they check his drug levels, etc. He will be admitted on Tuesday the 18th for two days of Cytoxan®, have a rest day on the 20th, and receive his marrow late in the evening of the 21st.

Brian had a transfusion this afternoon to raise his platelet count in preparation for his surgery tomorrow. This evening Mark took us out for my birthday for seafood and then we went out for ice cream.

This woman from BMT-talk, my Internet mailing list, read my complaint about not being able to find Shabbat candles, found me some and dropped them off at the clinic for me. She isn't even Jewish! Man, there are some wonderful people in this world.

It occurs to me as I read over my chronicle of the day that there is an odd juxtaposition of clinical scary stuff like chemo and germ-free living with total-

51

ly normal stuff like my birthday and ice cream. I think when I imagined what this would be like it was almost like an alternate universe. No vestiges of real life would exist, and we would be in Marrowland, which, I think, is somewhere in New Jersey. It's hard to believe the transplant is just ten days away and the world is still turning. How weird.

Tomorrow is a very long day, so I'd better sign off. Thanks to everyone who sent me 87 trillion e-mails for my birthday — it's nice to feel so loved at such a distance.

naomi

Date: Wed, 12 May 1999
Subject: Day -9: My husband — part man, part machine

Brian got up at 5:30 this morning and reported to the hospital, accompanied by his father, to have his Hickman placed. His father accompanied him because, unlike me, Joe actually is often conscious at 6 AM. We knew having him here would come in handy. The surgery was done under local anesthesia with sedation and Brian doesn't remember it at all. It took about an hour, and he was home by 10, feeling sore but pretty good.

I haven't actually seen the catheter yet. Brian hasn't gotten past the "ookey" feeling about it to really look at it. The pictures I've seen remind me of the show "Star Trek: Deep Space 9." There are bad aliens called the Jem Hadar who are born addicted to a certain drug and receive it through these white tubes in their neck and chest.

Brian had his first blood test through the Hickman today, and, ookeyness aside, is glad not to be getting stuck anymore. We will go tomorrow morning for training in how to change the dressing and flush the catheter, which has to be done at home.

Brian and I went for a class in food safety this morning. The center has done a fair amount of research on which foods are really dangerous and which ones aren't, so they are somewhat more lenient than many centers about Brian's diet. In fact, there are relatively few foods that are flat-out not allowed no matter how they are prepared: blue cheese, for example, and lox (a real loss!). Most foods are OK if they are cooked well. They are, however, extremely picky about how food is prepared and how to keep the kitchen clean. We have to change the sponge weekly and clean it in bleach solution daily; wash the outside of fruits even if we will peel them, including bananas; throw out leftovers after 2-3 days, and thaw frozen foods in the fridge instead of on the counter. Because of these restrictions, we have to ask that people not send gifts of homemade food to Brian. He can't have outside food when he's in the hospital at all, and when he's out of the hospital we can't vouch for how things were prepared. All in all we feel that the diet will require vigilance but not be overly burdensome.

Some other things that Brian needs to be careful about are more burdensome. He is officially off diaper changing for a very long time. In honor of this fact, Eve has decided that diaper changes are absolute torture and that she will hurl herself off the changing table in protest. So, although Brian can't change her, he is making himself useful holding her down.

The rest of the day was spent puttering around the apartment, eating yummy chocolate cookies I got for my birthday, finally getting the sewer line that was backing up in our house in Pittsburgh snaked and taking a nap!!!!!!! It's unbelievable how tired I am, and the fun has not yet even started.

We also had a visit today from a local Rabbi who works with patients and families. Hopefully, he will be available to us during this process so I don't

53

have to rely on the chaplains at the center. I'm sure they're great people, it's just that I need someone who speaks the same language religiously as I do. The Rabbi and his wife took an immediate shine to Eve, and she threw stranger anxiety to the wind so she could try to eat his wife's pearls.

Brian probably won't appreciate me telling you this, but tonight he announced he wasn't sure he was going to do this. He can't imagine the thought of starting as he is now, feeling quite healthy, and intentionally doing something that will certainly make him very sick and possibly kill him. He said he didn't think he could force himself to swallow the busulfan pills. Even an IV would be easier, and we know how Brian feels about IV's. He feels that, by going through with the transplant, he may be intentionally depriving Eve of her father while she's growing up. He pointed out that, if he didn't have the transplant, he'd probably live long enough for her to remember him.

We talked for well over an hour about this. I know I can't make him do it, but I also know it's the right thing to do. Still, I, too, hope that we can wake up from the nightmare and not have to do it. There's still a piece of me that thinks it might miraculously get better. It got better in January, why not now?

In the end, I told Brian it was his choice and that I couldn't and wouldn't make him do it. But I also said that, if he didn't have the transplant, Eve would spend the next couple of years hanging around the treatment room at the clinic, waiting for Brian to get platelet transfusions. In the end, he would still die and she still wouldn't have a father. He told me I was a tough lady. I think that's a compliment.

naomi

54

Chapter 3:
The Show Must Go On

Date: Thu, 13 May 1999
Subject: Day -8: Information Overload

Let the games begin.

This morning, Brian and I went to the clinic for our "teaching" with the nurse about his Hickman catheter and his chemo.

Some of you have asked for a better description of the Hickman (apparently the Star Trek references were a tad obscure). Essentially, Brian has a long white tube coming out of the middle of his chest. If left to its own devices, it dangles down near his navel. It splits into two tubes toward the end. Of course, it doesn't get left to its own devices. Brian wears it clipped to his medic alert necklace, or he can tape it to his chest or clip it to his clothing.

Care of the Hickman has many steps but is not overly complicated. First, the dressing is removed. Then, the area around the site where the Hickman comes out of his chest is cleaned with iodine and alcohol. Then, the outsides of the tubes are cleaned with alcohol. Then, a "split" gauze is placed around the exit site and a regular gauze is placed over the exit site, and the whole shebang is taped down. There is a slightly easier dressing he can use once the incision from the catheter insertion heals. The catheter also has to be flushed once a day. When he has blood tests they will do this for him, so we don't have to worry about it until he is out of the hospital.

I will get some supervision changing his dressing tomorrow, and after that we're on our own. Frankly, this doesn't seem appreciably worse than giving myself injections for our fertility treatments (or him giving me injections). You do what you have to do.

After we got our marching orders on the Hickman, we started in on the medications. As Brian begins his chemotherapy, he must take a variety of drugs that combat the side effects of the chemo and that fight various types of infection. His medication schedule for the next four days is literally round the clock. First drugs are at 7 AM, last at 2 AM.

Busulfan, his first chemo agent, is given in 2 mg tablets and the initial dose is geared to his size. So, being a big dude, Brian gets to take a whopping 42 tablets a dose. Now, don't get too excited, mind you, because they put these tablets into capsules so you don't have to take all those pills individually. However, there are only five tablets per capsule, so he still winds up taking nine capsules for each chemo dose. Those are given every six hours, and the dose will be adjusted each day as blood draws reveal whether he has the right amount of the drug in his system.

In addition to the busulfan, he must take:

Dilantin®, to combat the seizure side effect. Three big doses tonight, then one smaller one a day for the next four days.

Kytril®, an anti-nauseal, twice a day. This drug costs close to $40 a pill.

Acyclovir, an anti-viral, to prevent HSV (cold sores) and varicella (chicken pox) from becoming active as his immune system conks out. Twice a day.

Itraconazole, an anti-fungal, to combat aspergillus, a really nasty fungal infection. Brian is participating in a randomized study of this drug versus the more commonly prescribed fluconazole. For that reason, he gets the itra for free. It is a liquid taken three times a day. His report after his first dose is that it tastes really nasty.

Bactrim® and Cipro®, antibiotics, twice a day each.

Ativan®, Compazine® and Benadryl®, as needed for nausea.

Oh, and don't forget his multivitamin and his mouth rinse!

Of course, each drug has a rule about whether it is taken on an empty or full stomach, so the entire day is scheduled in terms of when he can eat. In the meantime, I get to play pharmacist, dispensing pills and keeping track. Also, if Brian should vomit after a busulfan dose while we're at home, I get to take a look and see if any whole pills came up so he can replace them. Eeeew.

By the time we were done going over his medications, we had missed half of the nutrition class we had planned to attend. The nurse was not overly concerned. I can take it another week, and Brian can read the caregiver manual and talk with the dietitian. So we came home for a break and then went back to the clinic for "Managing Care at Home." This class talked about managing symptoms at home and knowing when to call 911 and when to call the clinic and when to just let them know at your next appointment.

By the end of the day, we were totally overwhelmed with information. We figure that we are relatively intelligent people and that we should be able to manage all of this, but it is a lot to worry about. Frankly, I think you have to be reasonably intelligent just to figure out that you don't actually understand all of this.

My parents arrived this afternoon and we had dinner at their apartment. They are thrilled to see Eve, who seems pretty thrilled to see them back. We are grateful for some more pairs of hands to help out and for the company and moral support.

Tomorrow's another long day — I think they'll all be like that for awhile. Thanks for listening.

naomi

Date: Thu, 13 May 1999
Subject: From Brian

I've generally stayed out of the e-mail update business, leaving that to Naomi, but today I realized I wanted to say something to each of you who are following me.

In approximately nine hours, I will be sitting in the infusion room of the ambulatory clinic, looking at 42 pills of busulfan. I will then pick up and take, with my own hands, drugs which start me down a path from which I cannot turn away, no matter what.

As I have been contemplating and coming to peace with all of this, a few song lyrics have come to hold a great deal of meaning for me, capturing both the feel of the moment and what I hope to carry with me as I begin this journey. I'd like to share them with you:

>The show must go on...
>The show must go on...
>I'll face it with a grin
>I'm never giving in
>On with the show!
>   —Queen

Brian

Date: Fri, 14 May 1999
Subject: Day -7: On with the show

One day of busulfan down, three to go.

Brian woke me up just before 7 because a) I needed to get in the shower and b) he was in a panic because he had forgotten, during his shower, to cover his catheter with these lovely plastic-wrap-like squares that are supposed to keep his dressing dry. He was totally freaked because his dressing was wet. He called the clinic and they were unconcerned, but Brian was clearly agitated. The "loading dose" of Dilantin® he took last night was very obviously affecting him, and he was complaining of ringing in his ears, a common side effect. The exit site of his catheter was dripping a little blood as well, which made us both nervous.

He took an Ativan® to try to calm his nerves a little, and we headed up to the clinic at quarter to 8. Frankly, he was so loopy at this point that I was nervous about him walking into traffic! I don't think it was so much the Dilantin® as it was his nerves driving him to distraction and the Ativan® desperately trying to send him to a happy place.

We got there, checked in at the infusion room, and sat. And sat and sat and sat. And then we sat. After much shuffling around, it turned out there was some confusion over when he was supposed to take the first dose.

At about 8:10, I donned gloves (because the chemo is dangerous to me), counted Brian's pills for him (he was still pretty loopy), Brian picked up the first capsule, looked at it, held it up, said, "On with the show!" (an obvious line) and popped it down. This whole ceremony made me feel like I was being useful, which I clearly was not.

Shortly after he took his first dose, Moreen stopped in to see how we were both holding up. I think, honestly, that she was making sure we hadn't chickened out. It was nice to feel that someone was aware that this was a big moment and showing some concern beyond Brian's vital signs. Everyone else, including me, is a little more focused on transplant day. But for Brian, today was the point of no return.

Brian had blood drawn today at 8:30, 9, 9:30, 10, 11, 12, 1, and 2. This was to track the amount of busulfan in his blood stream. As it turns out, he apparently had very high busulfan levels in his blood stream today, and they cut his dose for the next four doses from 84 mg to 64 mg — ten less tablets, two less capsules.

Brian had very little ill effects from the busulfan today. He found the first hour after each dose a little queasy and is tinkering with various amounts and types of anti-nausea drugs to control that. We expect the nausea will get worse over time, but it may not.

While he was still having his blood draws every half-hour, the nurse supervised as I changed his Hickman dressing for the first time. She said I get a gold star (really, she did!). I'll have to do that every time he showers for as

58

long as the line is in, except when he's inpatient and the nurses do it for me.

Brian and I spent the morning watching Bullwinkle on TV and talking. My parents came and stayed with him for a while and then his father came while I went home and spent some time with Eve. Eve and I came back in the afternoon and she had a quick visit with him, and then I stayed with him through his 2 o'clock busulfan dose and a brief appointment with the nurse before we came home for the afternoon around 3. Even by 3 in the afternoon, the day felt like it had been very long and, frankly, anticlimactic. If this is the point of no return, shouldn't there be some kind of ominous background music or something?

Trying to figure out who is supposed to be where, when, is just about impossible. I have to keep in mind Eve's schedule, Brian's schedule, the health of all four of our parents, me, Mark and Eve as well as all of our personal preferences. It's like a gigantic logic problem. If John is not married to Mary, and Betty lives next door to a carpenter, who will sit with Brian during his busulfan days?

This evening we had a relatively quiet dinner at home, where I took my first real crack at preparing a meal following all the food safety guidelines. Brian usually does most of the cooking, and there is a reason for that. I am pleased to say that the food was at least edible. Brian was feeling pretty out of it and was blaming it all on medications rather than on tension and lack of sleep.
The high point of the meal came when he tried to cut his lamb chop with a butter knife, since we don't have steak knives. This would be hard for anyone. Brian managed to dump his whole plate on the floor. I knew it could easily have happened to anyone, including me, but it made him feel completely non-functional. If you know Brian well, you know that "non-functional" is not a state he's terribly comfortable with, so this was really hard.

The wonderful person who found Shabbat candles for us (we used a pair tonight, as you might expect), also baked us challah for our Shabbat dinner. She is so amazing! I actually got to meet her briefly today. She even looks nice.

Well, it's time for bed. Brian has to take a busulfan dose at 2 AM. The nurses told us to set an alarm, and we will, but setting an Eve is almost as reliable!

More tomorrow — on with the show!

naomi

I've been reading over the last few days' updates, and I have to say that I seem to have totally lost my sense of humor. I could just send out a daily e-mail that says, "I'M REALLY TENSE!!!" and it would have the same effect. I'm sorry.

I guess in yesterday's update I made Brian seem sicker than he really feels, so I should tell you right off the bat that, as I write this, he is making dinner. So, as you might guess, the nausea isn't too severe. The hardest two things about the last two days have been getting up at the crack of dawn and trying to eat dinner at the right time so his stomach is appropriately empty for his 8 o'clock dose of busulfan.

Brian is getting into the swing of this chemo thing. He finds the hour right after each dose the hardest — not really nausea per se, but rather a kind of full feeling in his stomach as his gut tries to deal with the toxic waste he has just swallowed. He takes Ativan® proactively before each dose to try to combat that fullness, which makes him spacey and sleepy.

For the hour after each dose, he wants someone with him but doesn't want to talk or do anything. After his 8 AM dose, I played solitaire while he spaced out in his chair at the clinic. After his 2 PM dose, he slept in the recliner. Eve kept toddling over and patting him on the head — at 6'4", his head isn't readily available to her very often. When he started snoring (and I mean snoring) she started clinging to me. Daddy was making scary noises!

At the clinic today, they gave Brian two units of packed red cells because his hematocrit was pretty low. Once his red cells were done, he and Mark went for a walk around the neighborhood. Brian's hematocrit and hemoglobin have been well below normal for a while, and his body has adjusted to having to do more with less oxygen. As he puts it, it's like he's been living in Mexico City for a year. Well, today's transfusion brought him back down closer to sea level, and he had a lot of energy. Mark said he had trouble keeping up.

They are dropping Brian's busulfan dose to 60 mg for the next four doses. Brian says he feels so good he's afraid they aren't giving him enough. The nurse says lots of people say that. The nurse assures us that many if not most people tolerate busulfan pretty well if they stay on top of the nausea with proactive meds, but it's hard not to feel like we're waiting for the other shoe to drop.

My inspiration for the day is a little boy named Michael whom I met in the infusion room today. He is on day +33 for his second transplant for leukemia. He is four. He and his mom have been here since his first transplant in February, and he was inpatient for 86 days. Now, a lot of you, particularly those who don't know kids who've had BMT's, might be thinking, "poor kid, to

60

be so sick and so little!"

Well, I don't know Michael well, but he sure looked pretty good to me. He had a big smile and was playing away, joking with his mom and the nurses. He had the best set of toys I've ever seen — I want a coloring box like that — and you would never in a million years guess what he's been through just by looking at him. Which, I think, goes to show you that, in this situation, the ability to live in the moment and base your attitude on how you actually feel, not where you've been or where you're going, serves you very, very well.

Please remember that we cannot have any flowers anywhere near Brian, so please don't send flowers to either of us. Someone sent me a card today with violets from their garden in it. It was a nice thought, but there was something of a panic when I opened it in the infusion room and the flowers spilled out onto the floor. No flowers means no flowers. Balloons, silk flowers, cards, toys, and mostly your warm wishes are very much appreciated.

naomi

Date: Sun, 16 May 1999
Subject: Day -5

Today was definitely a harder day than yesterday. Brian spent much of last evening with a sour feeling in his stomach — heartburn coupled with a belching hiccup. I kept hearing this sound coming from our bedroom and was sure he was throwing up. I'd go running into the bedroom, only to find him merrily e-mailing away, hiccuping as he went.

We did the usual drill at the clinic — blood draws at 8, 9, 10, 12 and 2. After the last blood draw, Brian sent me and Eve off to the park and went back to the apartment with our friend Mark.

At about 2:35 my beeper went off with the "I need to speak with you within 10 minutes" code from Brian. Since I don't have a cell phone out here and I didn't have change for the payphone, I piled Eve into the car and booked back to the apartment. In retrospect, this was probably more due to my own panic at seeing the code than any real emergency. I could have gotten change at any store in the area, but I sensed that I wasn't where I should be.

I was greeted by Mark at the door, with Brian saying in the background, "I blatted." In the entire time I've known Brian, which is about ten and a half years, he has vomited exactly once prior to today. Before that, he says he thinks he was maybe four the last time he threw up. So Brian has to feel pretty crappy to throw up. I, of course, felt horribly guilty for not having been there. First of all, it messed up my "perfect caregiver" image and second of all, pawing through Brian's barf looking for whole pills to report to the clinic was not exactly what Mark had in mind for a Sunday afternoon of fun and entertainment. There were no aforementioned whole pills, which was good because it meant Brian didn't have to take any more chemo to replace what came up.

Brian was feeling a lot better by the time I got there, and hopped into the shower. Mark played with Eve while I helped Brian with his Hickman dressing. As we started to clean the exit site, it started to bleed. It had oozed a little the last two times we changed the dressing, but nothing big so nothing to worry about. This seemed much worse, at least at first. It was less of an ooze and more of a drip. Frankly, I freaked. The heretofore simple, easy medical situation had gone haywire twice in one afternoon, which was two times too many for me.

I went to call the clinic, but called the wrong number (OK, I think of Sunday afternoon as "after hours." They don't.) I had to be transferred twice before I finally talked to a very calm nurse who was not very concerned but said to come in if I thought we should. I said we were on our way and went back to the bedroom, where I found Brian merrily changing his own dressing. The bleeding had stopped. So I called the clinic back (I knew the right number this time) and explained that we weren't coming after all. They just said, "Keep us posted. You did the right thing," which was nice because I felt like an idiot for going to pieces over very small things.

62

Meanwhile, poor Mark was trying to entertain Eve and answer the phone, which was ringing off the hook. Brian was starting to feel a little woozy again, and I was totally overwhelmed. At this point, I realized that everyone was exhausted. So, after Mark left, I called Brian's mom, who came over and put Eve down for a nap while Brian and I conked for an hour or so.

At 6, I woke Brian up to eat dinner, and he was feeling really out of it. Then we discovered the hot dog buns were past their expiration date — and looking it — and had to send his dad out for more buns. It was not a banner evening. However, after dinner Brian managed to do some dishes and play with Eve, which helped me remember that, although he is feeling yucky, he will probably not die in the next 24 hours.

As I write this, Brian has held down his 8 PM dose and seems to be doing a little better. He was more aggressive with the anti-nausea meds before this dose, and that may have helped. He is also wearing my "Sea-Bands." These are accupressure wristbands to help with nausea. Do they work? Who knows? It reminds me of the old gag — "Why do you have a banana in your ear?" "To keep the alligators away." "There aren't any alligators around here!" "See, it's working!" So, he'll wear them because they certainly aren't going to hurt and he'll take what works, placebo effect or no.

Today was upsetting if only because it shattered the illusion that this is going to be easy. It's not that today was so hard, it just wasn't trivial. We liked trivial better.

naomi

It's amazing what the right combination of modern pharmaceuticals can do.

Yesterday, Brian was just plain green in the afternoon, even after the "blat" incident. This morning he had a 9 o'clock clinic appointment, and we all thought he might keel over at any moment. Although he hadn't "blatted" since yesterday afternoon, he was looking quite ill and was complaining bitterly about the taste of the water. That's not so weird given how bad tap water can be. The thing is, he was also complaining about the taste of bottled water and was actually gagging on it. Chemo sure does interesting things to your taste buds.

Anyway, after talking to the doctor and nurse and discussing the cocktail of anti-nausea medications he was on, they decided to give him an IV shot of Ativan® in addition to the Compazine® and Benadryl® he had taken himself. Within two minutes he was a different person. A sleepy person, but a different person nonetheless. He slept a lot of the morning but clearly felt much better, and took Ativan® with the Compazine® and Benadryl® before his afternoon and evening busulfan, which really seemed to do the trick. He also thinks the accu-pressure bands are helping. There aren't any alligators around, either.

Now, don't get me wrong. Brian did not feel terrific today. However, he didn't vomit and he was somewhat functional when he was awake. In the late afternoon, we went out for a walk in the rain. We wound up at Rite Aid, where Brian found himself walking through the food section going, "Oooh! Pringles! Doritos, I could go for Doritos. Mint cookie ice cream!" He reminded me very much of a pregnant woman — almost everything looks bad, but you gotta have the things that look good.

Tomorrow, Brian will be admitted to the hospital for two days of Cytoxan®, a day of rest, his transplant, and maybe 4 weeks or so of recovery. We bought him one of those pre-paid long distance phone cards so he doesn't have to use his calling card every time he calls home. He will also have the computer and an electronic putting green, as well as assorted Legos. What can I say — he likes to plan ahead.

The amusing moment for the day came while the nurse at his clinic appointment went to get his IV Ativan® and I took a look through his chart. I like looking through the chart because it gives me a bigger overview of what's going on and also a peek at what the doctors are thinking, just in case they aren't sharing everything with us. In Pittsburgh, his chart says things like, "Brian Zikmund-Fisher is a delightful 29 y o male with history of thrombocytopenia." I told his nurses that they had to be nice to him because he was delightful — it said so in his chart!

Anyway, one of the things I found in his chart was the write-up from our first meeting with Moreen, our social worker. It was generally complimentary, but in the conclusion section she described him as "stubborn" and us as having "issues with control" which might be points of contention with the staff. I was fairly offended. I mean, we're doing the best we can here, and under the cir-cumstances we're doing pretty darn well! I then remembered the part of that social work meeting where she asked us to describe ourselves and we said we were "stubborn control freaks." Guess you can't blame her for writing it down.

We had a little scare mid-afternoon when Eve was with my mom and my mom fiendishly removed a piece of paper or some such thing from her mouth, causing her to cry at the top of her lungs. When I walked into the room, I saw that her nose was running, and she felt a little warm. I took her temp, and, sure enough, it was 100.0 rectally, which translates to about 99.0. "Great, she's getting sick, just what we need," we thought. We even went so far as to call the Red Team nurse to find out if they wanted Brian to be separated from her. Several hours later, when she was still happy as a clam and quite cool with no sign of a runny nose, it occurred to me that there's nothing that makes one's nose run and one's temperature rise slightly like a good screaming and crying fit.

It will undoubtedly take us a few days to get into the rhythm of inpatient life and of life at home without Daddy, but I hope to keep writing daily or at least every other day. Please remember that what I write is my impressions at a given time during the day. By the time you read them a lot can change, as those of you who called to commiserate with the barfing Brian found out today.

naomi

Chapter 4:
Riding the Second Wave

Date: Tue, 18 May 1999
Subject: Day -3

Brian checked into the hospital today shortly after eight. They have a one nurse per two patient ratio on his floor, and Jack Sarfaty of Internet fame was the other patient. I popped in and said hi to Jack in the morning. He looks good! Jack is on day +4 from his mis-matched unrelated BMT for chronic myelogenous leukemia.

Brian's nurse gave us the nickel tour of Brian's room and how everything works. We spent some time ironing out some kinks in the transition from outpatient to inpatient. They didn't have him down for the right study drug and they hadn't ordered a blood draw even though his platelets were low yesterday. Minor stuff, but it makes me glad that we stay on top of these things.

Rounds came by at about 9 and we waved at the hordes of medical folk who had come to gawk. There must have been at least 15 people there. Brian says he feels like it's feeding time at the zoo, and he's the ape. They didn't actually do much during rounds today because he's new. The docs came back later in the day to talk to him, but took so long getting there (a promise of "around 11" became "after 5") that I wasn't there when they came.

This snafu made me feel a little nuts. I want there to be a System with a capital "S" through which I can navigate. I don't like "we'll get there when we get there," because I can't be there all the time. Many caregivers spend 24 hours a day, or close to it, at the hospital on the BMT ward, but that just isn't feasible for me. Brian says he doesn't want that, anyway. As he put it, "I don't want you around 24 hours a day when I'm in a good mood. Why would I want you around that much when I'm sick?" But I hate the feeling that something important could happen at any time and there's no way to know when or what it will be.

They hooked Brian up to hydration through his Hickman and then he went for a walk. About ten long laps of the nurse's station is a mile, and he was out for a power walk, mowing people down with his IV cart. He was feeling very good this morning — better than any of the busulfan days and probably several days before that!

We ran into (pretty literally) Moreen in the hall and she did a few laps with us and explained some things about the schedule on the floor. This walk was kind of funny because Moreen tends to "dress up," unlike the nurses here, who dress down, and it was quite a site to see her matching Brian stride for stride in her heels. She confirmed, to my dismay, my belief that not much besides rounds is scheduled, so it will be somewhat random whether I'm there when Brian gets poked and prodded.

Brian had a huge lunch (shrimp cocktail, taco salad, Dove Bar and lemonade) and pronounced that he really likes this "whatever you want, whenever you want it" menu. There are many times coming when he won't want to or be able to eat at all, but he's enjoying it while it lasts.

Brian started his Cytoxan®, the second chemo drug, today. He got one dose today and will get another tomorrow. He also had a platelet transfusion. The major side effect of Cytoxan® (other than hair loss and nausea) is hemorrhagic cystitis — bleeding bladder infections. So, in order to avoid that, they give him tons of fluids IV and also irrigate his bladder. They inserted a Foley catheter today and he is now being "hosed" 24 hours a day. I think it is safe to say that having the Foley is not the high point of this experience from Brian's point of view. Seeing him lie in bed in a hospital gown for the first time doesn't boost my spirits, either.

Brian did OK with his first day of Cytoxan®. He was somewhat nauseated in the afternoon, but they drugged him up and that seemed to help.

I met some of the families on the hall. There's a kitchen, bathroom and lounge for families that we can use 24 hours a day, and families can talk to one another there, since visiting from room to room is a no-no. All of the Intensive Care Unit (ICU) BMT patients are on Brian's floor, so there are a lot of families in very rough circumstances around. It's really nice to see how everyone supports one another.

I talked for a while with a teenage girl, Devorah, whose father, Steve, is on day +1 for his transplant. I was struck by how matter-of-factly she was able to discuss her father's health. I guess I surprise people with how straightforward I am about Brian, too, but it's just odd to see that someone has had their transplant and still not been transported to Marrowland. There may still be life after day 0. There had better be.

After we left Brian, Eve and I went home to play and hang out and we both had nice naps. Then we went out to dinner with my parents, where my daughter, the vacuum cleaner, polished off two entire skewers of satay chicken. Now we're home alone and missing Daddy very much. This is going to be hard for both of us.

The big discovery for the day is that Eve adores having her hands washed, which is a good thing since she has to do it 8 zillion times a day. Brian's room sink has foot pedals for the water, and Eve thinks the faucet is just about the coolest thing ever.

There was one really nice moment today. Around 10, Barb brought Eve up to the hospital to nurse and brought a FedEx package with her. It was a recording our friend Michelle had made (on her kids' Fisher Price tape recorder, so not high quality) of the song she wrote for us. We listened to it while we set up Brian's room. It's still a tearjerker the second time around.

naomi

Date: Wed, 19 May 1999
Subject: Day -2 and Nothin' to do

Let me begin the update for today by telling you how yesterday ended. I finished writing my update, brushed my teeth, washed my widdle face, and went to get my jammies, which were tucked under the covers. When I pulled back the covers . . .

There was a large fuzzy teddy bear with a card from my brother and sister-in-law and their kids. The card said, "This was the fuzziest, shnuggliest bear we could find. Hope he helps a little." They had sent him to my in-laws, and my mother-in-law had tucked him into my bed while she babysat for Eve. He helped rather a lot, actually.

Brian's day today began with another do-see-do around the question of his nausea medications. He felt . . . OK . . . but not great. Finally, after a milligram of Ativan® and some Benadryl® and some droperidol, he was in a much happier place but very tired.

He managed to get down a bowl of frosted flakes, milk and berries and about half a cinnamon roll, but that and a 7-Up slushie was all he managed today. If he's not able to eat more, they will begin him on total parenteral nutrition (TPN). TPN is all his nutrition given IV, as opposed to the sugar water most IV's contain. "Steak and Eggs in a bag," as many folks call it. We're not there yet, and they're waiting to see what happens to his appetite now that he's done with his chemo (hooray!).

Brian was very restless this morning. Because of the catheter, it's really hard for him to get up, so he's been sitting in bed for 24 hours. The nurse thought she already heard some differences in his lungs from the sitting around, so he's been playing more with his breathing machine. This is a tube you inhale from slowly to raise a float on a gauge. The idea is to try to expand your lungs by forcing yourself to take deep breaths. As of yesterday, he was hitting the top of the gauge. We thought maybe they should install a bell so he could win a big stuffed animal or something. But today he was having a harder time. He has announced that, once the catheter is out tomorrow, he will be trying to walk 3 miles every day. That ought to keep his lungs in shape!

Anyway, Brian was trying to find different positions he could get into while still in bed with the catheter, which, coupled with those leave-nothing-to-the-imagination hospital gowns, resulted in some amusing sights for me. He finally managed to do some push-ups in bed. It's a good thing there isn't another building out his window, because he was mooning something fierce. The exercise made him feel a lot better before he decided that, in fact, he was really more nauseated than he thought, and he asked for more meds.

He hasn't felt like doing much since this morning and I've been being a noodge to get him to play on the computer or watch TV or listen to music — anything to be less of a lump. He brought tons of stuff to do, but he doesn't feel much like doing it. It seems like that's mostly the sedative effect of the drugs,

70

but it's hard to know.

It's difficult to tell whether I should be noodging more or less. I want him to do things. Somehow, as long as he's doing stuff, nothing bad can happen. You never hear of transplant patients dying while playing computer games. I know it doesn't work quite that way, but it feels like it, and it's hard to know where the line is between giving good encouragement and being a pain in the rear.

We had a visit today from his donor search coordinator, who brought the blood work report from all of the potential donors he tested. If you've ever wondered what $52,000 of blood work looks like, ask and I'll send you a picture. Now, if only the insurance company would decide once and for all if they're paying for it. Don't get me started.

I went back to the hospital briefly this evening and found Brian having difficulty opening his mouth. It seems that, although his nurse said they "always" give droperidol with Benadryl® because "many" people are allergic, they gave him droperidol by itself and his whole body went pretty much nutso. He got the rigors and his mouth clenched up to the point where he couldn't talk.

Before I got there, the nurse gave him some Benadryl® to calm the reaction, but when I arrived he was still clenching away. I was sort of miffed that no one had called the nurse when the Benadryl® hadn't worked, but then I guess his parents and Mark don't really know how fast it's supposed to work. I forget how much additional knowledge I've gained in the last year or so.

After another shot of Benadryl® he was doing better mouth-wise but very jumpy and having trouble with sensitivity to light. This was very scary to everyone around him. It was the first sign to all of us that "gee, he's actually kinda sick now, ain't he?" I left the hospital with Mark just after this incident, and Mark was visibly shaken. He's kind of a stoic type, so seeing him shaken is really unusual. It occurred to me that most of my shakiness is now just inside — it's too much a part of me for it to be visible anymore.

I called Brian late this evening, and he seemed to be doing somewhat better. Tomorrow is a "day of rest," meaning that he gets no treatments or therapies, just his antibiotics, antifungals, antivirals and antinauseals if he needs them. This conflicts with my definition of rest, which would definitely include a pina colada.

Eve is having a difficult time with the changes and tension around her. She isn't sleeping well at all and she is very clingy to me. She slept better at birth than she does now. I feel horrible about this, of course, because I want to spend more and better time with her. But then, I also want to spend more and better time with Brian. She does love seeing Brian in the hospital and has enjoyed walking along the hall on his floor and banging on the picture windows.

There is no right answer, and hopefully she will adjust as the month or so that Brian is inpatient continues. I had a long talk with Moreen about trying to strike this balance. I simply don't know how much time away is too much. It seems like any time at all is too much. This is a very unfair burden to place on a little kid. And, frankly, it's not too much fun for her mother, either. Moreen assures me that Eve will still know I'm her mother even if I'm away for most of the day, but it's hard to believe that in my heart even if I know it in my head.

Thank you to all for your concern and prayers. Please understand that we are not always able to return your calls and messages right away, but that they mean a lot to us none the less.

naomi

Date: Thu, 20 May 1999
Subject: Day -1: Blatman returns

Brian seemed much better when I came in this morning. When rounds came around, the attending said, "OK, you did great. Wanna yank out that catheter now?" I actually thought Brian was going to do it himself, and Dr. S. must have too, because she said, "Wait until we leave. They need to deflate the balloon." (There's a little balloon that they inflate inside the catheter to hold it in place). She also noted that under no circumstances was he to get the antinausea medication that gave him such a nasty reaction last night. Geez, I didn't even go to med school and I figured that out.

As soon as the catheter came out, Brian took a shower and put on his own clothes. That seemed to make a big difference in his mood, as you might imagine. Unfortunately, his stomach was still giving him some trouble all day, but it seemed to be improving as time went on. He finds himself very torn between getting meds for his nausea and toughing it out so he can stay more alert. It comes and goes and so does he.

Brian walked 21 laps, for a distance of over two miles, today. In other words, he walked more than I did. Laps are how you get to know the other patients on the hall. Patients aren't allowed to socialize with one another since they don't want one person getting some bug and then spreading it to the whole ward, but they can talk as they pass in the hall. This makes for very limited conversation, but you make do.

On today's walk we walked behind Steve Cohen, Brian's next door neighbor, whose daughter Devorah I met in the kitchen the other day. Steve is an Orthodox Jew, and we had a good giggle about the fact that, from a distance, it looked like he had shaved all of his hair except a circle on top. Just as we were contemplating why anyone would do that, we realized he had shaved all his hair, and was wearing a yarmulke. Steve thought this was pretty funny, too.

We also walked in opposite loops with Jack Sarfaty and a man named Pedro who, as far as I know, speaks no English. Everyone has their own way of getting into the groove of walking, but everyone's determined to walk, walk, walk! It's frankly the people who aren't out walking who I worry about.

Although his stomach was still flipping on and off, there really wasn't any doubt that Brian was doing much better. I brought Eve over late this evening and he immediately sat up, picked her up, and started tickling her and playing on the bed. This was a marked contrast from yesterday, when I basically had to force him to hold her at all. It was a moment of great relief for his wife. I can do this, just as long as he keeps being himself most of the time.

Brian told me today that he didn't feel much like talking on the phone. He felt like concentrating on himself and just getting through. I, on the other hand, want to talk. A lot. It's not that I'm desperately sad or miserably lonely. I just need a lot of reminders that I'm not alone. The apartment is very empty at night. Eve isn't sleeping very well. Things go bump. There's no one to wake up to (OK, no one taller than three feet). I see Brian at the hospital but I don't feel like I can lean on him. He's got his own stuff going on, in case you hadn't noticed. And that's hard because he's my best friend and the one I usually talk to.

Then, of course, there are my parents and my in-laws. But my in-laws have a whole different issue here: it's their kid. And it's hard to know how to be together in this without getting into a whole weird turf battle about Brian. The trouble with my parents, on the other hand, is that, if I ask for help, I feel like I'm surrendering my adulthood. It's hard to let my mom take care of me without feeling like she's, well, taking care of me. I know this experience should be drawing us together, but so far it just seems to be bringing up all the old baggage. Don't get me wrong, I'm glad they're all here and they're all being really helpful. But when you've lived hundreds of miles away from your parents and in-laws for as long as Brian and I have, being close together isn't easy.

Ah, now, that feels better. See? I want to talk. You know the number. Tomorrow is the big day. His marrow is supposed to arrive around 9:30 PM, but since it's coming from Australia one presumes there may be some delays.

Several months ago, I corresponded with a fellow BMT caregiver about the need for patience as we waited to schedule Brian's transplant. Patience is not my strong suit. I shared with him my thoughts about the Jewish custom of "Counting the Omer." This is a tradition where you count the days between Passover (the exodus from Egypt) and Shavuot (the giving of the Law at Mt. Sinai). Of course, the Israelites didn't know how many days to journey. Now we know to count 49 days, so it almost seems pointless. We could just mark it on the calendar. But by counting their days, as they must have when they wandered in the desert, we remember that every day brings us closer to the goal, even if we don't know exactly how long it will be.

I find myself reflecting on that exchange because tomorrow, Brian's transplant day, is also Shavuot. Two years ago on Shavuot, we waited for the conception of our child and thought it would never come. Last year, Eve's due date was Shavuot, and I honestly thought she would never come. Tomorrow, again, as Jews around the world study late into the night to await the birth of the Jewish people, we will be waiting for Brian's rebirth. And then, of course, we start counting days all over from zero.

Oh, and, in a bit of poetic nicety, it is traditional, on Shavuot, to read the book of Ruth, the story of Naomi.

Chag sameach (Happy Holiday) to all, and many blessings.

naomi

Date: Fri, 21 May 1999
Subject: Happy re-Birthday Brian!

This morning was the culmination of a lengthy project I started the month before we left Pittsburgh. Unbeknownst to Brian, I arranged for his friends and family to put together a video for him to watch on his transplant day. People came to our friend Eleanor's house to tape their well wishes, gathered at Brian's department, or sent individual tapes that were edited in. People were instructed to do whatever they thought would be "appropriate" for someone who probably wouldn't be feeling well on a celebratory occasion. It was interesting to see what people's warped ideas of "appropriate" were.

My brother and sister-in-law told everyone to sing "I'm a Little Teapot" on the tape, so there was kind of a running gag that included numerous renditions of "I'm a Little Teapot" by people ranging from business school professors to seminary presidents. My brother sang it in Ubby-Dubby, a language they used to do on the original ZOOM! TV show. My niece's fife and drum core played it on the fife, and a friend sent a riddle "worthy of the Sphinx" which began, "I am a vessel for caffeinated liquid. I am small in stature, neither am I slender."

Brian was fairly sedated while he watched, but he really enjoyed it. A few moments actually caused a guffaw to cross his lips — my brother's Ubby-Dubby version, Nancy's riddle, one of his professors yelling at him to "Get up! Quit lying there!," and his family doctor and friend Bill Mitsos' impression of Marvin the Martian. Brian commented on how nice so many people's wishes were. Thank you so much to everyone who participated. It was fantastic. And, believe it or not, he was actually surprised. I can't believe we even came close to pulling this off!

Brian had a great day. He walked over three miles and felt very good. The weather was gorgeous and you could see the mountains from his room. After putting Eve to bed, I headed over to the hospital with Brian's mother to be with him at the big moment. The nausea had dissipated and he was feeling terrific but very impatient, as you might imagine. We had a silly fantasy about the cooler going around and around on a luggage carousel at the airport with a sign nearby that read, "Many Marrows Look Alike. Please Check the Luggage Tags on Your Marrow."

At 9:35 PM, the transplant coordinator walked onto the ward with a cooler containing four big bags of marrow. She was accompanied by a very tired Australian doctor. The marrow sat in the room on the counter, awaiting final approval to transfuse from the blood bank. We had fun reading the label and figuring out what time it must have been collected (and which way does the international dateline go? Is it tomorrow or yesterday? Help!). We figure it was about 30 hours from harvest to transplant, which may explain why that doctor was so tired! We put on Michelle's recording of the song she wrote for our going away party, and all three of us cried.

At 10:40 they finally got final clearance to start infusion, and away we went. Brian turned on his "Attitude Tape," a mix of music he picked out to help him through this whole journey. As the marrow made its way down the tube into his Hickman, the strains of "Fanfare for the Common Man" came over the speakers. It was something.

Happy re-birthday, Brian!!!!

Praised be our Eternal God, Ruler of the universe, who has given us life, and sustained us and brought us to this time.

naomi

Date: Sun, 23 May 1999
Subject: Day +1

At the beginning of today, Brian was not the sickest person in our family. Eve woke up vomiting at 3:30 AM. May I say, for the record, that dealing with baby barf is at best a two or possibly three person job. By this evening, she was running a mild fever and coughing and sneezing a lot. So, for the duration, Brian is without his little "pumpkin."

Eve flatly refused to go back to bed after her barfing, and I finally wound up with her in the living room in the dark, looking out into the night at the beautiful lights. It was actually quite peaceful — an oasis of sanity in a crappy situation. Eve seemed to calm down a little, and I said, "Look, Eve, it's nighttime. Everyone is asleep except for little girls. Can you go to sleep?" She put her head on my shoulder and went right to sleep. Pretty cool.

Because Eve was sick, I did not make it to rounds this morning. My mother went instead, which worked out just fine. After some miscommunications, failures to tell me things, and general frustration on my part, I put a notebook in Brian's room so anytime anything important happens medically, whichever of the various parents are there can write it down. Then, when I get there, I don't have to feel like I missed something important.

Some mild side effects of various sorts have begun to crop up for Brian. He has a slight rash on his left side. It is so minor that he didn't know he had it until the doctor asked him how long it had been there. No itching or anything. The doctors feel it is probably a reaction to an antibiotic he is taking, but that, given how mild it is, it's not worth changing at this point.

Brian's blood pressure was up a little today. This may well be a reaction to the cyclosporine, and they are watching it to see if he needs blood pressure medications. This is pretty normal for people on cyclosporine, and not cause for great alarm.

Brian's nose started running in the last 24 hours. This might be an allergy or a very early stage of mucositis. It doesn't seem to be an illness of any kind, but they may order a CT of his sinuses just to be sure.

While Brian was receiving his dose of methotrexate this morning, one of the medications he is taking to prevent GVHD, he felt a pain in his lower ribcage area. They stopped the injection and then started it up again very slowly, but the pain didn't go away. The doctor poked and prodded him and proclaimed that it wasn't anything really scary like air in his Hickman, but that he wasn't sure what it was. Most likely it was gastrointestinal, which made sense since Brian's diarrhea is back and he had a bout right after the pain started.

Still, all in all, Brian was feeling good today. He walked a total of 20 laps. Mark, who walked the last ten with him, asked to be given time to stretch before his next workout. He had a visit from Cindy Prichard, the wife of another MDS patient here, and from a distant kissing cousin of mine who lives nearby.

However, this evening, Barb called from the hospital to say that Brian had vomited rather a lot including a fairly sizeable amount of blood. They poked him and prodded him and quizzed him about everything he did today. They checked his platelets and hematocrit and decided to give him another unit of platelets even though he probably doesn't need it just to be sure. He doesn't seem to be bleeding internally. They did some blood cultures but don't expect to see anything. The official diagnosis is he "irritated his gut." They stopped the Lomotil® he was taking for diarrhea so that anything yucky will go out the bottom rather than the top and told him to limit his roughage.

I can't begin to describe how helpless it feels to get a call like that. Something is wrong, we don't know what, you can't do anything about it, and you're not here anyway. I know that these calls will probably get worse before they get better, but that doesn't mean I have to like it.

When Barb left the hospital, Brian was doped up from the various antin-ausea medications and sawing wood big-time. Eve is busy not sleeping next door. It's going to be a long night for all of us.

naomi

Date: Tue, 25 May 1999
Subject: Day +3

I didn't compose an update yesterday for two (related) reasons:

1) I was home all day with a touch of a tummy bug and didn't feel much like writing and

2) I was home all day with a touch of a tummy bug and didn't see Brian.

My day yesterday stunk. Eve was still sick and barfy and grouchy and not sleeping. I started with the runs around 6 AM. Joe came over to take care of Eve so I could sleep. I started to feel better by lunchtime but Eve's nose continued to run. I, of course, wanted to go up to the hospital right away, especially given Brian's previous night's blood barfage, but didn't want to risk giving my tummy bug to Brian. Of course, there was always the possibility that he already had it, and that's what had caused the original barf.

However, yesterday, Day +2, was an outstanding day for Brian. He actually walked 50 laps — 5 miles — and ate 2900 calories. This for someone whose appetite is supposed to be waning and energy flagging.

Today was similarly an excellent day. Good appetite, little or no nausea, no fever, no mouth pain. His greatest complaint is a gassy heartburn type feeling that doesn't respond to antacid, suggesting it might be mucositis in his GI tract. However, he is eating fine on top of it and it doesn't bother him much.

His bilirubin (a measure of liver function that can indicate veno-occlusive disease or graft vs. host disease) was ever so slightly elevated Sunday, which alarmed me but bothered his docs not at all. They aren't even going to check it again before tomorrow. Dr. S. told me not to worry. She said, "I'll tell you when you need to worry," which was funny but not terribly reassuring. They do this stuff hundreds of times a year. I hope to do it only once in a lifetime. I'll worry if I darn well feel like it!

Although we are, of course, pleased he is doing so well, there is a feeling of waiting for the other shoe to drop. I said this to someone on the phone today and Brian picked up a shoe and dropped it. Our friend said, "No, Brian, the other shoe." So then, of course, he picked the other one up and dropped it. Very predictable!

Brian is spending his time watching TV, walking, talking on the phone, walking, playing on the computer, walking, eating, walking, and even doing a little dissertation work. Oh, and he walks a lot, did I say that? At this point, the doctors just laugh as he goes plowing by on his laps. And when I say he walks, I mean aerobic power walks.

His favorite time for this is during rounds. First of all, he believes it's important for his doctors to see him out and about so they think of him as a person and not just a body and a chart. Second, the docs congregate in enormous

79

hordes in the hallway during rounds, and Brian loves plowing through them and making them scatter. I have dubbed this "bowling for doctors." His Fellow has started sticking out his foot to trip Brian as he goes by.

Today during rounds, Brian had to ask his attending physician for special permission to bring in plain Hershey Bars. Seems you can get Snickers, M&M's and Reese's from the hospital food service, but not plain Hershey. And you have to get special permission to bring in outside food. This request rather tickled the assembled masses, and his doc OK'd it only on the condition that he share.

Brian said he feels more relaxed than he has in months. He says his only job in the hospital is to get better. As long as he is feeling good, this is essentially a mini-vacation in a rather strange and not terribly posh hotel with decent room service.

I'm back to the hospital each morning, but Eve still can't go. I'm not sure they've been separated for long enough for Eve and Brian to really miss each other, but that's coming soon!

For those of you who know or are concerned about Jack Sarfaty, I saw him this morning doing laps. He's been in isolation due to respiratory symptoms for several days. This means he wasn't allowed out of the room and everyone who went in had to wear gowns and gloves and masks. I don't know how he felt about it, but it put the whole rest of the floor in a blue mood. Jack was out today. He looks great, and it was good to see him after so many days of isolation.

naomi

Date: Wed, 26 May 1999
Subject: Day +4

Brian says he feels like he's slowing down, but given how fast he was going already, that just means he's doing great instead of terrific. Yesterday he only walked 43 laps, down from 50 the previous day. Oh, horrors! During rounds he told the doctors that only 40 of these laps were actually aerobic, and everyone just had to laugh at him.

Because Brian is doing so well, seeing him in the hospital isn't as hard on me as I thought it would be. We actually get more quiet time together now than we do when everything's "normal." I sit around and do crossword puzzles, he watches TV or reads or sleeps or whatever, and we both get our exercise together. If it weren't for that pesky IV and the threat of death hanging over our heads, this might be an enjoyable respite. I know, picky me.

Brian has the first real signs of mucositis today. The back of his mouth feels, as he describes it, like he burned his mouth on pizza three days ago. It doesn't hurt, but the skin feels like it's been flayed a little. He also has a sort of heartburn/gas feeling, not really pain but not comfortable, in his esophagus. All of this is much to be expected. He's still eating like a champ calorie-wise, but has changed what he's eating some to accommodate the discomfort.

Pedro, one of Brian's frequent walking "companions," went into ICU on a ventilator. The rumor is that his mucositis is so bad it actually closed off his windpipe. This is terrifying. Pedro was out walking laps one day and was on the vent the next. If it could happen to him, it could happen to anyone. And I'm married to anyone, if you catch my drift.

I stuck my head in to Steve Cohen's room today and we talked about Pedro. I know I'm not supposed to visit room to room because they don't want caregivers tracking whatever bug might be about to declare itself in one patient and introducing it to another. I did it anyway. Sue me. Steve says Pedro's situation has made him much more determined to keep up with all the mouth rinses and whatnot they have you do for mucositis. Frankly, we're all scared.

Eve still has a cold, but seems to be generally on the mend. Brian misses her and I think, if she knew enough to know it, she would miss him too. As for me, I'm just taking one day at a time and trying to keep my head above water.

As you might imagine, this whole situation is a logistical nightmare. Someone has to watch Eve while I'm at the hospital, and I'm still trying to actually, you know, live some semblance of a life. Just getting the laundry done or the garbage taken out or the groceries bought is hard because I have to tote Eve along with me. I have all these people who are here to help, but somehow the things I need help with never seem to jive with anyone's schedule or mood. And of course, by the time I realize I really need help with something, it's often too late. Everyone wants to be helpful, but, in the end, what would be helpful is having Brian home. I know it could be a lot worse, but I don't see it as a contest. Just because my life isn't the worst possible doesn't mean I have to like it.

Thanks to all for your words of encouragement, and we'll see you tomorrow!

naomi

Date: Thu, 27 May 1999
Subject: Day +5

Brian walked a mere 4.2 miles yesterday, and we are all, of course, very concerned.

Yesterday afternoon his temperature started creeping up and he was feeling sort of warm and blah. Come to find out (no one tells me anything) that they had reduced his hydration yesterday because he was drinking so much by mouth and they didn't want to stress his kidneys. But yesterday he didn't drink as much and it seems he got slightly dehydrated. Today, they upped his hydration and he's feeling much better. His blood pressure, however, is still pretty low which is of some concern. A few days ago it was too high, now it's too low. You can't win.

Brian's mouth is starting to show more mucositis signs. He has a sore throat and his mouth has white "scalloping" on it. The scalloping is caused by old cells that aren't getting sloughed off like usual. He is still getting all of his nutrition and a fair amount of hydration by mouth, however, and the nutritionist yelled at him to start eating more protein.

One of the big issues for Brian right now is that food is losing its taste. He discovered today that sucking a lemon didn't taste even vaguely disturbing to him. He is drinking a lot of Gatorade because the slightly salty taste is appealing.

Steve Cohen and his wife, Sharon, stopped by the room today on their walk. Steve's mouth is really starting to bug him, and he's having trouble talking. We shared with them that Brian, in preparation for his transplant, taught himself some American Sign Language so he could talk when the mucositis got bad. Sharon said that they didn't know any ASL, but Steve proceeded to suggest a number of amusing gestures for how he was feeling. At least he still has a sense of humor.

I find it difficult to establish really how well Brian's doing compared to the norm. Obviously he's not doing badly, but everyone at the hospital is so hell-bent on the mantra "don't compare yourself to other patients" that it's hard to get a sense of how much of the bullet he has dodged/is dodging/will dodge. I know I should just be taking things one day at a time, but I spent the whole last year gearing up for the worst and hoping for the best, knowing that a long road lay in front of us. Now we're on it, and I'm still prepared. I just want to know how much is behind us.

I am continuing to do the "head above water" thing. My mom was going to come over to help me get the laundry done this afternoon but didn't feel well and so didn't make it. I know I shouldn't be mad at her for that. I know she isn't sick on purpose. But somehow I want everyone else's life to stop because mine has had to. It's hard not to feel like it's all just a big excuse not to help with my laundry. Not that I'm paranoid or anything.

I am very conscious of the fact that I am never alone save when Eve is sleeping and the 10 minutes each way when I walk to the hospital. Twenty-four-hour caregiving shifts are rather tiring. It's funny how the time when Brian has left me "alone" is the time it turns out I'm the least alone I've ever been in my life.

Eve is on the mend but still has a runny nose. She did, miraculously, actually sleep last night, waking up only once. I'll take it! I lost count at 9 times two nights ago.

naomi

Date: Fri, 28 May 1999
Subject: Day +6

This morning, we mowed Brian's head again. He still hasn't lost his hair and he was getting a little fuzzy. We have discovered that when you shave your head and then let it grow out all one length, your head looks something like a koosh — you know, those little balls with the rubber hairs coming out from all sides.

The doctors at rounds were all giggling because yesterday, after the nutritionist noodged him about eating more protein, Brian ordered and ate four hard-boiled eggs. Let's just say he follows directions. Except when he's being stubborn.

Dr. S., his attending, is a very powerful presence and teases Brian a lot. You may recall that last week I asked her something and she said, "Don't worry about it. I'll tell you when to worry." Today I asked something, she told me not to worry, and I said, "Oh, I'm not worried. You made it clear I'm not to worry without permission!" This cracked everybody up, including her.

Today I was feeling really miserable and tired at the hospital. Brian and I had a long talk about what might help me feel better. I said one of the problems is that, by the time I get home and eat lunch, it's Eve's naptime so I don't get to see her much. Brian pointed out that the same hospital service that delivers his food will, for a fee, deliver food to me in his room. That way I could have lunch while I'm still with him and free up my former lunchtime to spend with Eve.

I nixed this at first. I said it was too expensive. Which caused Brian to give me the look you give someone just before you slap them for being so stupid. Sure, $20,000 in unreimbursed medical expenses we can handle. Just don't splurge $5 on lunch. Perspective is a wonderful thing. I'm glad Brian is still able to give it to me, because obviously I've totally lost it.

So Brian tucked me into his bed, got out the wooden-roller-massage-thingy someone had sent and rubbed my feet. Then we ordered lunch together and had a little picnic. It was very relaxing for me, although I felt a little silly having this guy with an enormous infusion pump attached to him take care of me. Which one of us is sick?

Speaking of which, in the middle of this his nurse came in and asked why I was in bed. I made the mistake of saying I was "not feeling well." She went white. It took some doing to convince her that I wasn't contagious, just grumpy and tired, and that I promised on 87 bibles to not come to the hospital if I was sick.

More tomorrow, and tomorrow, and tomorrow!

naomi

Date: Sunday, May 30, 1999
Subject: The Memorial Day Curse

Yesterday, the folks watching our house called to say that someone had broken in and stolen our stereo and VCR and rifled through everything else. Luckily, everything of true value to us either has no value to anyone else, is in the safety deposit box, is with us, or is a "you have to know what you're looking for" type of piece (e.g. antiques belonging to my grandfather). And our TV is too big to transport easily. They didn't take our tape deck because they know junk when they see it.

The people living in our house were understandably very shaken. I, on the other hand, just started to laugh. What more could possibly happen to us? From our point of view, this is more of a pain than anything else. We'll have a new stereo in place by the time we get back to Pittsburgh and, unlike our sub-letters, this doesn't make us worried about the bad guys coming back in the night to get us.

Ain't life great?

naomi

Date: Mon, 31 May 1999
Subject: Day +9 and feelin' fine

Over the weekend, Brian's attending commented, "We've had several people eat through transplant. But never quite this . . . much. We're going to charge you extra for the food."

Brian is doing great. I mean really great. I mean, it's just totally uncalled for how great. I am typing this sitting on his bed in the hospital while he plays this boxing video game with Mark. I, as a caregiver, feel totally extraneous to his recovery experience. Indeed, sitting around while he plays video games with Mark is, well, pretty typical activity for me even when he's not in the hospital.

He moved today to a bigger room. Room 909 was previously occupied by the legendary Jack Sarfaty, who was discharged on day +16, so this is a lucky room.

To deal with Brian's mouth, they hooked up a PCA pump (patient controlled analgesia, a morphine pump where he pushes a button to get a dose when he needs it) for last night, but he didn't use it. Thus far he's just used a topical anesthetic and I don't think he's even used that much.

He's feeling like he can eat more solid stuff, which is good because he was running a risk of turning into a fruit smoothie. Every morning the doctor says, "another day or two and we'll start TPN," and Brian just smiles. I think he's still eating out of sheer stubbornness.

Brian's hair is . . . loose. If you pull on it, little bits come out, but it's not falling out of its own accord at all. He's getting pretty irritated with me pulling on it all the time just to see it come out. I look like a chimpanzee grooming its young. Can you tell we've gotten a little wacky here at transplant central?

Oh, and for those of you concerned, I'm thinking of writing a book entitled, "How the Lord Backed Up My Plumbing and Let Me Sleep." First, my e-mail was down yesterday so I napped while Eve napped rather than write an update. But I was still tired. Then, when I was getting ready for bed, I noticed that the disposal in our kitchen had backed up into our bathtub. This is a truly disgusting sight. Actually, my first thought was that someone had snuck into the apartment and vomited into our bathtub. They have weird burglars around here. So my morning shower was out of the question, and I slept in today. I'm feeling a lot better, and thanks for your concern. They fixed the plumbing while I was at the hospital this morning, so things are looking up all around.

naomi

Day 10, nothing to report, thank you for tuning in, goodbye.

Seriously, Brian's still doing just great. He is having increased pain in his feet from the cyclosporine he takes to combat graft-versus-host disease, so he's cutting back on his walking. Yesterday, I think he walked like two and a half miles. Practically nothing. He is also getting blisters on his feet, and his doctor told him to take it easy on the walking for a while.

Brian also had a little tiny bit of nausea today. It was kind of funny, because he was sitting on his bed, eating an English muffin, going, "I feel nauseous." Crunch, chew, chew, chew. "Maybe I should take some Benadryl®." Crunch, chew, chew, chew, gulp. "I don't feel too good." So, as you can see, it was truly incapacitating. He was also really tired and the Benadryl® made that worse, so I left him a little before 1 o'clock sawing some wood.

The Transition people stopped me in the hall today to say that his parents and I need to take the "pump class" so we can learn how to work the infusion pumps he'll be taking home with him. They were optimistic that he'll be sprung soonish and want us to definitely take the class this week. It's hard to share that optimism when his blood counts are still at bottom, but hey, they know better than I do.

Actually, his counts are not completely at bottom, and may even be going up. The docs want to see the trend over the next two or three days to be sure. I stopped our favorite nurse in the hall and asked her if I could whisper the "e-word," engraftment. She said I could whisper it, just not to the docs. It's funny — one of the reasons we picked this center was that we felt like they were very up front and straightforward about what we could expect. The flip side of this, however, is that they never want to tell you anything unless they're pretty sure. And when you're reading the tea-leaves (or, as the case may be, the blood count leaves) for signs of engraftment, it's frustrating that they want to be so sure before they make a pronouncement.

At the beginning of the day, it looked like poor Eve was finally going to get to see her Daddy. But at 10, my mom called to say her nose was dripping again so the visit was off. This put me into a major funk. I think the separation has, in some ways, been harder on me than on either of them. When Brian can't see Eve, it's just another reminder that things aren't right. It also plays directly into my major fear of being a single parent. And, selfish as it may seem, I think I need Brian to see her so he can tell me what a great job I'm doing with her. Last night I brought Brian a video of Eve cleaning all the pots out of the cupboards and generally being cute, which he greatly enjoyed. I miss being a family together.

Of course I had to take this bad mood out on someone. This someone happened to be the nurse Brian had today, someone I didn't care for to begin with and certainly don't care for now.

The transplant floor has a general policy that neither patients nor family are supposed to look at the patient's chart without having a member of the staff with them. They can't legally prevent us from looking at all, but they don't want us looking by ourselves lest we read something that we misinterpret and freak out. I can understand this, actually, given the way they phrase things. For example, instead of Brian's chart saying, "Patient has no pain," it says, "Patient denies pain." Which you could take the wrong way, I agree. But on the whole I think this rule is silly — if I have a question I'll ask it, don't you worry!

Anyway, I went into the hall to check the results of a liver function test, came back in, told Brian the results, and the nurse said, "Remember, you're not supposed to look at the chart without me!" Big mistake. Huge. This was not the thing to tell a nosey, information addicted, grumpy wife! So I let her have it, which I think caught her totally off guard. Mental note to self: Do not kill nurses. Nurses have great power over life and death of husband. End note.

In the afternoon I went out by myself (remember that?) and had a massage, a present from Brian's mom. I needed it. I could probably have had two or three.

Ms. Eve is gearing up for the big oh-one on Saturday, and with any luck at all we'll have the party at Brian's room. (Shh, it's a surprise, she doesn't know!)

naomi

Date: Wed, 2 Jun 1999
Subject: Day +11: Reunited

This morning, as the doctors were coming around for rounds, Brian cued up Queen's "Don't Stop Me Now" on the CD player and set it playing as they came in. It was very funny to us, probably not very noticeable to them. But you gotta figure that when he has time to think of these things and feels up to doing them, it's pretty close to time to go home.

Brian continues to eat like a horse. The nutritionist who just rotated onto the floor told me she hasn't met any of the patients and doesn't know any of their names, "But I know your husband eats 2700 calories a day." They took away his PCA since he wasn't using it. Merely having it in the room for two days was apparently sufficient. He appears to have a mild infection in his Hickman — no fever but some tenderness — so he's on yet another antibiotic.

The big news of the day is that Eve's nose has slowed down to the point where the hospital staff feels that she can safely visit. Right now she's having her afternoon nap, and then she's off to see Daddy!

Brian's mother and I took the pump class today so we can do Brian's plumbing for him when he comes out of the hospital. Sharon Cohen sat next to me in class — apparently Steve is going to be sprung very soon, too. We also learned how to flush the Hickman line, and I was amused at how easy it is for me to draw flushes into the syringe, get the air bubbles out, and otherwise deal with the medication bottles. Two years of infertility treatments make you pretty handy with a needle. Nice to know it all had a positive purpose, aside from the obvious one asleep in the crib in the next room.

It's unlikely that Brian will be sprung before the beginning of next week and possibly much later than that, but now we're ready!

Now, if you'll excuse me, I have to go devour more of the two dozen rumballs from my favorite bakery which a friend shipped me from Pittsburgh.

Life is good.

naomi

p.s. Last night, as I was in a truly foul mood, I put on a favorite CD and listened to my own personal theme song, which I have adopted for this adventure. Eve and I danced and we listened to it about 100 times. It was very therapeutic. I thought I'd share the lyrics with you:

"Bagels with Angels" by Susan Piper

I had bagels with some angels
In a deli on the mainline Sunday morning.
It was impromptu.
They don't flash their halos
And there weren't any wing flaps
They don't throw their weight around the way they used to.
All in all the morning was quite laid back.
When the conversation dragged I took a chance and asked
What are the advantages of waking up an angel?
It must be very different when you're dead.
And the one who looked like Jerry Lewis said,
Well,
We can fly in the face of fear.
We can ride that second wave.
We can laugh in the face of God.
God wants us to laugh.
God knows we can be brave.
We can hold somebody's hand.
We have thrown our shame away.
We can fly in the face of fear.
God wants us to try.
God knows it's not too late.
We can ride the second wave.

This was just the sort of answer
You'd expect to hear from angels.
It was just a little holier than thou.
Onions and tomatoes
Are the stuff my life is made of.
I should ask them something practical for here and now.
They could really put away the coffee.
Listen fellas, what would you do if you were like me?
What are the advantages of waking up a human
In a world I think would kill me if I let it?
And the balding heavy set one answered,
Don't you get it?
You can fly in the face of fear.
You can ride that second wave.
You can laugh in the face of God.
God wants you to laugh.
God knows you can be brave.
You can hold somebody's hand.
You can throw your shame away.
You can fly in the face of fear.
God wants you to try.
God knows it's not too late.

You can ride the second wave.

I felt full and happy.
It was nothing like religion.
It was not the whitefish salad or the way they shook my hand.
It was just the combination.
Kind of freaky.
Kind of grand.

I can fly in the face of fear.
I can ride that second wave.
I can laugh in the face of God.
God wants me to laugh.
God knows I can be brave.
I can hold somebody's hand.
I can throw my shame away.
I can laugh in the face of fear.
God wants me to try.
God knows it's not too late.
I can ride the second wave.

Date: Thu, 3 Jun 1999
Subject: Day +12: Go White Cells!

Today's rounds began with the attending uttering those five little words every BMT patient longs to hear: "Your graft is coming in." Believe it or not, they are actually talking about releasing him over the weekend, which would be day 14 or 15! His mom and I met with the transition nurse today to talk about outpatient life.

There is one catch, however, and today it turned out to be a doozy. He needs to be able to take all of his medications, except the antibiotic for the infection in his Hickman, by mouth. For the last two or so weeks, he's been getting them IV. So today, they started trying to switch the meds over.

Unfortunately, today Brian also felt much more nauseated than he has in a while, and he upchucked his first dose of oral cyclosporine this afternoon. I think he is feeling really discouraged by this. Just when they tell him he can go home, he comes up with the one symptom that would prevent it.

Of course, he is also concerned about what might be causing this nausea since it hasn't been bad up until now. It might be the last dose of methotrexate he got yesterday, but he's concerned that it is GVHD of the gut. That wouldn't be surprising, but it would be a royal pain. I think everyone has a type of discomfort that is worst for them, and for Brian it is nausea. He'd rather be in excruciating pain than nauseous. Unfortunately, he just needs to wait a day or two and see what happens.

I've been doing a lot of "last year at this time" thinking recently, since last year at this time I was past my due date and roughly the size of Montana. Last year yesterday, tornadoes hit Pittsburgh and Brian and I sat in the basement contemplating how dramatic it would be if I went into labor. However, the only water that broke was the flood that came through, punching a hole in our basement wall.

A year ago today I had an ultrasound and was positively sure it was a boy. I could tell myself just from looking at the screen. Turns out you actually do need medical training to distinguish and umbilical cord from a penis. Oops.

A year ago at this time we had no way of knowing what the next year would bring. Which is a good thing to think about, because we can't really know what this coming one is going to bring us, either. We just have to roll with it.

Best to all, and hopefully the news will be more unambiguously positive in the days ahead.

naomi

Yesterday afternoon and evening, Brian's energy level, and hence his mood, went down the toilet. He just felt horrible. They went scurrying around, trying to figure out what might be wrong, and finally told him to get a good night's sleep.

Morning brought more energy and appetite and a very unnerved Brian. He was quite literally freaking out when I got there this morning. He was sitting on the bed refusing to move. I called Moreen and she came right over.

There's nothing like being told you're going home to make you sick, but we may have some answers. First, Brian's magnesium level was really, really low yesterday. This is a common problem with cyclosporine, and can cause you to really drag. When they took it again today it was still really low, so it must have been super low yesterday for it still to be low today after getting some magnesium IV.

Second, Compazine®, the anti-nausea medication they gave him yesterday, is a bad actor for Brian. It seems to have made him very spacey and unable to function. Luckily, that's a temporary issue. No Compazine®, no problem if, indeed, that is the problem.

Third, and perhaps most significantly, his culture came back positive for c.Difficle, an intestinal bacteria. It probably caused most if not all of his diarrhea and possibly some of his nausea as well.

So Brian is going to start a new antibiotic today and see if we can't get this little bugger under control. In the meantime, he is in "contact isolation." This means that visitors must wear glove and gown, and if he goes out of the room he must wear glove and gown. He is allowed out of the room, can have the door open and no one has to wear masks, which is nice. We are trying as we speak to regroup in hopes of salvaging Eve's party tomorrow.

I must say, however, that it was rather alarming to be standing in his room this morning, minding our own business, and have someone roll up an isolation cart and start slapping stop signs all over the door without explaining it to us. It wasn't as bad as we thought (respiratory isolation is really the stockade!) but a simple "Hi, your culture came back positive, you're in isolation" might have been nice.

The good news is that, paradoxically, the isolation does not affect Brian's discharge from the hospital. They need to prevent other patients from getting this, but he can go out of the hospital with it. In fact, they'd like to get him out of the hospital to reduce the risk of infecting other patients. Brian's counts were steadyish from yesterday, and the big hurdle is still going to be getting his meds down orally. He is eating today, however, so that's a step in the right direction.

Ms. Eve had one terrific visit with Dad on Wednesday. She popped in on him briefly yesterday but he wasn't up for a visit. Today she was going to visit just as they put him in isolation, but we're hoping to bring her up later on for a visit in the hall.

Brian and I spent an hour talking with Moreen today — about how much this episode threw him for a loop, and about me wanting him home and feeling overwhelmed because I'm not the ideal, Martha Stewartesque homemaker who can make this all work without any problems. One of my big issues is feeling incompetent for needing so much help. There are single mothers all over the world who manage to get their laundry done, their groceries purchased and their garbage taken out without anyone helping them. Why can't I? Moreen said, "Naomi, you don't have to manage their lives. You just have to manage yours." This did not make me feel much better.

Add to this the fact that I've never had to deal with Brian's parents without him around before. It's not so much that they're so difficult, but rather that every family has its own way of doing things, and his family doesn't do things the same way mine does. If I need something done, I have to say it very explicitly. I have to stop saying, "Do you have any time to help me go grocery shopping?" and start saying, "I'm going grocery shopping at 3 and I need someone to come and help me carry the bags. Who is coming?" Brian usually does the translating for me, but he can't do that right now.

So, he's losing it and I'm losing it, each in our own individual way. The fact of it is, he's still doing really well. But even in the best of BMT circumstances, it's still a BMT and this situation is still really, really difficult.

Steve Cohen had an altercation with the food service today. He gets kosher food from the kitchen, which is a fairly restricted menu. Today, he ordered oatmeal and they sent up a packet of "quick oats" (not instant), a cup of hot water and a bowl. This was useless — you can't cook quick oats that way. So he called down and told them to just send up the regular oatmeal off the regular, non-kosher menu. They said they couldn't do that, because he's on a "restricted diet," and that he'd have to take it up with his doctor. He absolutely could not convince them that "kosher" was not a medical restriction, and that therefore, if he wanted to eat off the regular menu, it was none of his doctor's business. I thought he was going to explode. Ah, the joys of bureaucracy.

naomi

Date: Sat, 5 Jun 1999
Subject: Day +14: The BMT ward parties down

First, let's get the ucky clinical stuff out of the way.

Brian's nausea was kicking up a tad more this morning and his counts have been absolutely flat for three days. His wife was not happy.

We talked at rounds with his doctors about what might be going on. Option one is that all of his nausea is caused by a combination of the c.Diff and the Flagyl® , which he is taking for the c.Diff, and which, as it turns out, causes nausea. This is why I like it that the pharmacist attends rounds with the doctors. He can point out stupid stuff like this.

Option two is that Brian has some GVHD of the gut. In the interest of trying to figure this out, they are taking him off oral Flagyl® and putting him on IV to see if his nausea gets better.

I cornered Dr. S. in the hall this morning to talk about his counts and the fact that they aren't moving much. She reassured me that hanging out for a few days at the level he's at isn't bad — counts do all kinds of crazy things — and she talked more with me about GVHD and what her hunches are. She's betting the Flagyl® is the problem, but she said, "that's a soft bet." I really appreciated her taking the time to discuss this with me, even though she didn't offer a whole lot of new information. It helps me to see how she's thinking about things. It makes me feel more "in the loop."

By afternoon Brian seemed to be feeling a fair amount better, which was good because the social event of the year, Eve's birthday party, took place in his room.

Because Brian is in contact isolation, the nurses helped us plot and plan. Frankly, they seemed to really get on the bandwagon when I mentioned that, if we could pull this off, they could have the leftover cake. First, Brian's IV pump was isolated inside Eve's play-yard, so she could run around the rest of the room and we didn't have to worry about her pushing buttons or pulling on cords. His parents, my mother, Mark and I all gowned and gloved. Eve wore regular clothes but we stripped her down to her onesie before she left his room and changed her clothes in the stroller in the hall, leaving the "contaminated" clothes in Brian's room with his laundry.

Eve's cake (with a kangaroo for "Evearoo") was brought to the door very briefly so we could all see it, then sliced at the nurse's station (and of course, the extra was devoured by said nurses) and brought into Brian's room with some candy and candles. We forgot matches, so they were imaginary flames, which is good because Eve can't burn herself on imaginary flames. Eve danced to Peter, Paul and Mary, sat on Daddy's lap while he fed her ice cream cake, hung out while Mommy opened the presents for her and then watched an episode of "Bear in the Big Blue House" which Grammie and Grandpa had given her on video. Eve also tripped over some wrapping paper

96

and went headlong, getting a minor nosebleed. But hey, that's part of being a toddler.

Eve's favorite present by far was from Mark, who collected keys from his coworkers that don't open anything anymore. He strung them on a colorful key ring and gave them to Eve as a present. She's always playing with (and losing) my keys, and now she has a set of her own.

When we returned home from the hospital, there were several Happy Birthday messages on our answering machine, including a call from Bill Mitsos, a friend who is also one of the doctors who caught Eve a year ago. He said he was going to call at the actual time of the birth, but that he didn't want to get up at 5:04 AM, and he figured I probably wouldn't appreciate being woken up at 2:04 AM. It was a really nice touch to the day.

In fact, believe it or not, the whole day was nice. I remember that, when we arrived, Moreen told us that there would be times in this process when we just wanted to stop time and live in that moment forever. I thought she was crazy. I mean, hello, this is a life threatening medical procedure. But, in fact, today was one of those times. I doubt that, in all the birthday parties Eve has yet to come, she'll beat the joy and warmth of this first one.

In closing, I'd like to say that I know I do my fair share of kvetching (complaining) about what's wrong with this whole situation. And while I stand by those kvetches, I thought I'd share with you a list of things that are really pretty nice about it:

Starbucks raspberry scones
The view of the mountains out the hospital window
Eileen, one of Brian's nurses
Caramel Frappucino
My "call of the day" from Pittsburgh
Dancing babies
Bear in the Big Blue House
The city at night, as seen from our living room window
"Bagels with Angels" by Susan Piper
Rum balls from Pittsburgh
A rousing game of "where's Eve?" before bed
Snoodles the Bear and Ollie the Hippo, my bed companions
Getting to see Mark almost every day
Eve getting to know her grandparents
Brian's attitude tape
Eve at the park
Steve Cohen, who always talks about his health by saying "Thank God" and
    "God willing!"
Fan e-mail from all of you!

Thanks,

naomi

Chapter 5:
The GVH/Zoster Fiasco of '99

Date: Sun, 6 Jun 1999
Subject: Day +15

By day's end yesterday, Brian's appetite had pretty much returned. I went to the hospital this morning to find Brian eating a cheese, tomato and mushroom omelet, a bagel, some tea and some Gatorade. Wasting away, he was. On rounds, he told the doctors he really wasn't feeling 100%, and that his appetite comes and goes. Dr. S. reassured him that he only needed to be able to eat a little bit, and that she didn't think this was GVHD of the gut because it wasn't getting worse. They agreed to not change any more meds over to oral today and gave him the option of trying cyclosporine orally tonight.

I'm sitting there during this conversation thinking, "Wait a minute, they're talking like he's not eating, and yet I see that he's eating a lot. He's talking like he can't eat while he eats. Huh?"

Well, turns out that the nutritionist hadn't done Brian's calorie counts for the day prior to rounds. At about 12:45, Dr. S. opened the door to Brian's room and said, "2700 calories and 2000 cc's of liquid?!?!? I don't think that's GVH," and we had a good laugh. She gave us to understand that, if she had known how much he was eating and drinking, she would have pushed the oral meds more, but Brian is pretty glad she didn't. I think his largest obstacle is convincing himself that he can do this and not having a conditioned reflex against taking the pills. He hates being nauseous!

This whole thing frustrates me because there's a part of me that thinks Brian just needs to get over it. He just needs to decide he's going to take his pills and then do it. Brian doesn't see it that way. To him, there's something really wrong in his gut. But being on the outside and not privy to first-hand information, it always seems to me like he's being a little whiny. And then, of course, I feel guilty for thinking that. After all, don't you think Martha Stewart is a little more sympathetic to her loved ones? Probably not, actually.

Today was Dr. S.'s last day as Brian's attending. Dr. W. takes over tomorrow. In honor of her last day, we played a little "stump the doctor" with Dr. S. There are a number of questions we have that don't have any import whatsoever for Brian's treatment but which make us curious. For example, why do Brian's nails continue to grow while his hair is falling out? It seems that, not only do nails grow (although slower), but some hair rarely falls out (like pubic). Who knew?

As I was leaving the hospital, I spoke with her briefly in the hall and she said, "He's going home really soon." Echoing that, the charge nurse came into

Brian's room while he was having lunch and said, "You look like discharge material." I, on the other hand, will believe it when I see it.

Steve Cohen, however, is discharge material. In fact, he was discharged today. And while we're lonely without him and Sharon around, we're thrilled that he's doing so well. We'll all be out here for a couple more months, so I'm sure we'll see Steve and Sharon plenty in the weeks ahead.

I'm still hopeful Brian will be home in the next few days, but of course anything can happen. Someone asked me today when the doctors will consider that Brian is "out of the woods." Pretty much, I think the answer is never, although big milestones come at 100 days and 1 year. The longer he goes, the better that is. As someone once told us, "He'll never be out of the woods, but he'll probably find some nice meadows."

naomi

Date: Mon, 7 Jun 1999
Subject: Day +16: One step forward, two steps back

Last night, Brian managed to take his oral cyclosporine in liquid form. He kept it down, but he wasn't happy about it. This morning, when I arrived, he was looking pretty green. He ordered breakfast, ate a little, took his next dose of cyclosporine and, as one of the nurses put it, "hit the eject button."

After some discussion with Dr. W, the decision was made to go back to IV cyclosporine and give his tummy a rest for a few more days. He's eating fine, but the meds just won't stay down. Dr. W. thinks it may just resolve itself in the next three or so days, so we'll try again toward the end of the week and then, if necessary, do an endoscopy (stick a camera into his gut) to look for GVH.

The prospect of putting off the change over to oral medications was very disheartening to me. I need him to be moving forward, even in little steps. I don't like the feeling that he's standing still. When he entered the hospital, we never expected him to come out anywhere near this early, but, having let myself dream, it's hard to go back. I would be happier, in some ways, if he had been sick all along, his counts had never started to come up and I wasn't expecting anything.

I talked today with one of the chaplains who came around to introduce herself. The Rabbi who was assigned to us came by a few times to talk to Brian, but hasn't really been keeping in touch. I took this opportunity to collapse into a puddle. After all, puddle mopping is her job. Someone commented recently that there seem to be an awful lot of people around here who are just there for you to talk to, and I really think that is true. I have to stifle my natural urge, however, to say "fine" when these people ask me how I am. It's hard to avail yourself of help for your problems when you don't want to admit that you have any.

Anyway, the chaplain and I talked about how I was doing with all this and why the latest news put me into such a funk. Basically, I'm terrified that Brian will never come home. As long as he's getting better, even if it's slowly, I believe everything will be all right. But now he's going backwards and, even though he's just exactly where he should be or even better for this stage, backwards is backwards. As I sobbed on about this, the chaplain just sat there and said, "mm-hmm . . . sure . . . mm-hmm," which was really all I wanted. I just needed someone to listen to me talk and not say, "Gee, Naomi, you really seem to have gone around the bend."

I've taken to going downstairs for a little break each morning at the hospital. I sometimes get a snack or a coffee in the coffee shop and then stroll down the hall to the chapel. The chapel is a tiny and very beautiful space with lots of hard wood and flowers. I just sit there for a minute or two. Sometimes I pray for Brian, but more often I just enjoy the quiet.

On days I don't make it downstairs I sit in the "quiet room" they have set up on Brian's hall. It's a miniscule room, just big enough for two chairs and a coffee table, with a not terribly exciting view. But the solitude is nice, and it helps me collect my thoughts. It seems like I'm so busy taking care of things and asking questions and worrying that I'm not aware of what I'm really thinking until I take a few minutes to sit in the quiet.

Eve visited Brian twice today, and enjoyed being carried while he walked his laps. She popped another tooth and has decided to give up night-time sleeping entirely until her wisdom teeth erupt. So I'm a little tired. Just a tad. Which probably isn't helping my mood.

My mom went back East today, and Brian's mom is leaving on Wednesday for ten days. That leaves Joe and me to hold down the "hang with Eve" / "hang with Brian" caregiving fort. That won't be much of a change for me, but it means a lot more work for Joe.

I've also started to obsess about Eve's childcare for the fall. It seems unwise to put her into group daycare when I go back to work since Brian will still be very immunosuppressed. I'm going back to work, and we basically have no plan. I don't like not having a plan.

At this point, in my fantasy, a woman holding an umbrella floats through the air like Mary Poppins, lands on our doorstep carrying a carpet bag and all is right with the world. But it doesn't work that way. And, of course, this is exactly the sort of thing I should not be obsessing about because I can't do anything about it. But my personal motto is, "It's never too early to worry."

I got an absolutely astounding e-mail today. I can hardly believe it. One of the people who gets these updates regularly and has been getting them since the beginning e-mailed me and said, "I haven't had time to keep up with how everything's going, but I presume everything is fine." Now, don't get me wrong. I know that not everyone has time to read the volumes I'm putting out. That's OK. And I know this person's intention was to offer a friendly greeting. But honestly, this really hurt. And hurt was not what I needed given how I was feeling today.

First of all, I want everyone to read every word I write because every word is important to me. I know that's not realistic, but the reminder that I could write something so crucial and have it wind up in a friend's circular file is painful. And second of all, the notion that someone could presume everything is fine tells me that he really isn't clued into how lousy this whole situation is.

I'm taking this person off my mailing list. I don't know if that's the reasoned, mature thing to do, but it's what I need to do right now. I can't invite someone into my support system who isn't willing to stay informed about how things are going and support me through the reality of the situation, not just what he "presumes."

On the lighter side, my friend, attorney and godmother of my child, Michelle, had the following to say about my aspirations to be a Martha

102

Stewartesque caregiver:

"As for Martha Stewart, she doesn't do any of that homemaking stuff herself. She has an entire staff to do it. Plus, I have never seen an issue of *Martha Stewart Living* about caring for your BMT loved-one. However, if there were such an issue, I could just see the article now:

Isolation Can Be Beautiful

Many BMT patients find themselves in isolation when they develop certain infections. Regular, hospital issue warning signs posted on the hospital room door and entry way can be rather plain and unsightly and take away from the at-home feeling you've developed for your loved-one's room [see April issue, Decorating at Transplant Centers]. With just a few items you have lying around your house (or check with the nurse's station) you can turn those isolation warning signs into works of art.

Start with the standard five-inch stop sign post. Using a white glaze, tone down the bright red, giving it more of a glossy pink look. Then, using one-inch lace trim (I prefer Alencon, tatted by Mlle. Souci in Provence, see back of issue for contact information) tack gently along outer edge of stop sign. Be sure your glue gun is set to the low setting. For the rest of the warning signs, be creative! Mix and match colors and textures to complete the look.

You will also be given several hospital issue gowns to wear while in your loved-one's room. While you can't add materials to the gown, find other ways to accessorize, such as pearls with matching earrings, an antique brooch, pinned just so, or even a floral silk scarf [see March issue, Accessorizing Hospital Scrubs and Other Uniforms]. After that, use your imagination!"

Keep on truckin'!

naomi

p.s. I've been missing a lot of calls from home lately, which makes me sad 'cause I'd like to keep in touch. Being the neurotic person that I am, I tend to figure that if you call me and don't leave your number then you don't really want to talk to me. I know that makes no sense, but please bear with me and leave your number.

Date: Thu, 10 Jun 1999
Subject: Day +18 and +19: Mama said there'd be days like this

I want to begin by saying that everything I am about to write is absolutely true and has occurred in the last 36 hours. I could not make up a day like this if I tried.

Tuesday night, 9:00 Eve goes to bed

9:40 Naomi goes to bed. I'm really tired and figure if I go to bed early I'll get a really good night's sleep. (Note subtle foreshadowing)

Wednesday, 1:42 AM The fire alarm goes off. Eve and I dutifully evacuate the building. This yields several interesting observations:

1) White noise machines block an incredible amount of noise. Eve sleeps with one of these gizmos that makes a constant waterfall sound to block out street noise at night, and she did not wake up when the fire alarm went off.
2) Being woken up in the middle of the night and brought into a bright hallway where loud bells are ringing is about the most terrifying thing that can happen to a one year-old.
3) People under 50 get dressed to go out for a fire alarm. People over 50 wear their jammies and robes.
4) I don't dress like the rest of my age group.

2:30 Eve refuses to go back to sleep but is finally cajoled by her mom.

7:00 My alarm goes off and I toddle into the bathroom to discover there is no hot water. It seems that a burst pipe in the hot water system is what caused the fire alarm to go off.

8:00 I head up to the hospital.

9:20 We get Brian's counts. They're up. Brian is feeling kind of green but having much success with Ativan® to manage it, and doing a fair amount of eating. Operating theory is still that it's gut GVH, but if he can use Ativan® prophylactically to help him take his pills, they hope to release him Friday or Saturday. On the other hand, when have we heard that before?

1:00 PM I go home. Brian's mother left today, so his dad and I are the only caregivers. Joe is supposed to go up to the hospital around 2, but he develops a rash on his neck and wants to go to the family medicine clinic to get it checked out just in case it was something that could be passed to Brian.

Now, at this stage in the narrative, I'd like to pause and have you consider what would be about the worst thing that could happen that would not

104

endanger anyone's life directly. Be creative. Think about it before reading on.

3:00 PM Joe calls to say he has been diagnosed with shingles, a reactivation of the virus that causes chicken pox which attacks the nerve endings, often in the skin. This means that Joe can't be around Brian, Eve can't be around Joe, and Eve, since she's been exposed to Joe, can't be around Brian. We are up a creek. Here, Brian is about to be released to our care, and we won't be able to care for him and Eve at the same time.

4:00 The Infectious Disease department calls to recommend that Eve have her chicken pox vaccine today and start taking acyclovir (an antiviral) in six days. Before today, they had said not to have her get the chicken pox vaccine because it can cause low-level cases of chicken pox. This was fine with me since I'm not a huge fan of the chicken pox vaccine. But now they feel that, given the shingles exposure, she should go ahead and have it and take the acyclovir to combat any chicken pox she might get from it. They assure me repeatedly that, if we do this, Brian will not need to be isolated from Eve.

I take Eve to the family medicine clinic where they dutifully give her the shot and then inform me that they will not write a prescription for acyclovir because, "Brian has had chicken pox and is therefore immune. Plus, we aren't 100% certain Eve's been exposed." I'm sitting there thinking, "Well, we know she's been exposed now because you just stuck it in her leg, you morons! Brian isn't immune to anything, that's the whole point!" In fact, I actually say this, minus the "you morons" part. Nice to know I still have a very tiny bit of self-control. After several go rounds and another call to the transplant center, we agree to disagree for a few days until the results of Joe's blood tests come back.

I am now steaming, and do what anyone in my situation would do. Go to Starbucks and have a Caramel Frappucino and a raspberry scone. Much better.

When I get home, Brian calls to say that he has been speaking to Dr. W. who is a major infectious disease guru, and that Dr. W. feels that Eve should be isolated from Brian whether or not she has the vaccine and the acyclovir. At this point, I totally lose it. If it makes no difference in Brian's care one way or the other, where did they get off telling me to give my child a vaccine which I would not otherwise have used? That's a parenting decision. And although I can't control much in this fricking situation, I am still Eve's parent.

Shortly after 6, our volunteer family comes over to watch Eve while I take a shower. Bet you forgot about the water being off, now, didn't you? Well, they fixed it during the day. I then go up to the hospital to have a little chat with Dr. W.

Dr. W., Brian, and I have a rather pointed but quite productive discussion about the situation. Dr. W. feels that the risk of a new exposure to varicella zoster (the virus in question) to Brian is very low, but not zero. Therefore, he is willing to allow Brian and Eve to live in the same house, or at least sleep in the same house, if they limit contact with each other for about two and a half weeks starting early next week. Joe should be past contagion by Wednesday, so he'll be able to help out. Dr. W. also promises to help me get the matter of the acyclovir for Eve straightened out.

I express my extreme displeasure that this was not fully explained in the first place. Although we probably would have wound up in the same place, I feel I should have been given more information. He agrees, but points out that that was Infectious Disease's job. I say, "Yes, but they're not here for me to yell at." To his credit, he agrees that being yelled at is in his job description as attending.

Throughout this conversation, Mark is sitting on Brian's windowsill, trying to be invisible. After Dr. W. leaves, he says, "Man, I hope you're never mad at me. You're taking a shovel to the back of the man's head and he's totally defenseless because you're being so polite!" Nice to know I have some useful skills.

Meanwhile, back at the ranch, we still have a child care crunch. Eve can still come to the hospital through Saturday, but she won't put up with long visits. I contacted a local emergency nanny service, but they weren't able to provide anyone for today. They are working on tomorrow, and have found someone for Saturday.

Today, Eve and I slept in and then went up to see Daddy for an hour. Aside from that, he will be alone for pretty much the entire day, which I feel just horrible about. He is trying to take his meds orally today and tomorrow and hopefully will be sprung on Saturday.

I am delighted to report that Pedro has come off the ventilator. He was on it rather longer than I had thought he would be. It was my understanding that people who go on the vent for mucositis usually come off when engraftment starts, but Pedro stayed on so I guess there were some other problems. The whole floor seemed to be happy with the news of his improvement. The nurse who's been caring for him was beaming ear to ear, looking into his room as he watched a soccer match on TV, saying, "Doesn't he look great?" He sure does. Thank God.

So, that's where we are! I'm a little tense, as you might imagine, and not thrilled with what our living arrangements are going to be like for the next several weeks. But we'll manage, we always do!

naomi

p.s. I guess I made everyone feel guilty with my last message about phone calls. Sorry to all of you who called and paged yesterday whom I didn't call back. I'm working on it!

106

Date: Sat, 12 Jun 1999
Subject: Day +21: Naomi loses it

Brian's attempts on Thursday to take oral cyclosporine were, um, abortive. After two unsuccessful attempts with his day dose and one with his night dose, he declared loudly that the experiment was over. His mood was not aided by the fact that, due to the shingles crisis, I only saw him for about an hour and a half total all day. The docs said they'd have GI (that's the gastro-intestinal folks, not the army) look at him on Friday.

Friday, a nanny service finally came through with five and a half hours of sitting for us and I came to the hospital as usual. Rounds came just as Eve arrived for her morning nursing, and, given that we were paying $12 an hour for the privilege of me being there for rounds, I asked them to skip Brian and come back. They didn't make it to Brian until about noon.

They looked him over, discussed his gut, the darkening skin on his hands that is quite painful when he rubs it, and his elevated liver function test results. The working theory is that all three of these problems may be caused by a mild case of GVHD, so they ordered a skin biopsy, asked GI to come, and casually said, "We'll scope you on Monday." Mind you, we've been sitting around all week watching him feel green, and they've been saying, "We'll scope you at the end of the week." Now they can't scope him until Monday because of the weekend. Like they didn't know that a weekend comes right after Friday. Duh.

After the docs left, the nurse cheerily said, "Why would you want to leave? Your ANC is only 330?" Now, one might argue that it isn't prudent to leave the hospital with an ANC of 330, since you're still pretty prone to infection. But why would he want to leave? Um, I don't know. When was the last time you lived in a hospital for a month and had every bit of what goes in, out and on you measured and discussed? When was the last time you spent a month involuntarily away from your spouse?

Moreen, our social worker, was in the room when the nurse said this. She took one look at the expression on my face and politely but firmly asked the nurse to leave. Smart lady.

At this point, I totally and completely lost it. For those of you who know me well, take the most losing it moment you've ever seen and multiply by at least three. There was yelling, there was swearing, there was crying, there was more swearing.

Poor Moreen was directly in the line of fire. I was completely hysterical and taking it out on anyone and everyone, but especially on her. Here we were, having watched Brian for a week, all the while saying, "Gee, think it might be GVH, let's wait until the end of the week," and, as far as I could see, we were now saying, "Gee, think it might be GVH. Let's wait until next week." Not to mention that I have no child care arrangements past Saturday

107

and Eve stops being able to come to the hospital because of the great shingles fiasco, so Brian will be alone.

Moreen pointed out that there isn't a whole lot of difference from the doctors' point of view between "the end of the week" and "Monday." I know what she means, but my world doesn't have weekends right now. In my world, every day is exactly the same as the day before except that the counts move around some and Brian barfs more or less. In my world, a one-year-old and a twenty-nine-year-old both need constant care and I'm the only one to do it. In my world, having Brian get IV medications by day is fine if he just can come home and sleep right next to me at night. In my world, every day Brian is in the hospital is possibly another signal that he won't ever come home.

Of course, by now it was almost 1 o'clock and I had to go home because the sitter was leaving. Then Eve had her one-year check-up at the fine, upstanding medical practice that was still refusing to write her a prescription for acyclovir. The doctor, without my asking for any kind of assistance, helpfully suggested that if Eve was having trouble sleeping due to the changes in our lives and her feeling insecure, it would help her feel more secure, somehow, if I let her cry and scream all night. She also hinted that she thought it was high time I weaned Eve. I miss our doctors at home. They may not always agree with me parenting-wise, but they keep unsolicited advice to a minimum! I just smiled and nodded. No point in arguing.

On the way home, well, you can guess. Caramel Frappucino.

At this point I was at least calm enough to consider what the hell we were going to do since Brian wasn't coming home. After some brainstorming with Moreen, Brian and Dr. W., we came up with something of a plan. Dr. W. agreed that if we were going to treat Eve like she was contagious for chicken pox anyway, there wasn't any reason Joe couldn't start taking care of her again when our child-care ran out. He also agreed to wait until I could get there in the afternoons to examine Brian so I could talk to him and ask questions.

Meanwhile, back in shingles-ville, the family medicine clinic got around to saying that, gee, they weren't actually all that sure this was shingles, and they'd like to see Joe again (did I say we missed our docs at home?). The transplant center finally wrote Eve the acyclovir prescription themselves. They noticed that they had some prescription pads lying around, I guess.

So, clinically, here's Brian's situation. Platelets are stable (there's a phrase we thought we'd never hear!) and all other counts are rising. If his skin biopsy is positive for GVHD he'll start steroids today, if not they'll scope him on Monday and perhaps start steroids then. If his gut thing is indeed GVH, a very few days of steroids should have him out of here. But I'm done making firm predictions.

naomi

108

Date: Sun, 13 Jun 1999
Subject: Day +22

Well, it's one of those good news - bad news days.

Good news is, Brian's skin biopsy was negative — no GVHD of the skin.

Bad news is, Brian's skin biopsy was negative — he can't start steroids until they find GVHD somewhere, presumably his gut, tomorrow. It would have been useful if they had found something, because starting on steroids would also have treated the presumed GVHD of the gut, and he could have gotten out of here without the endoscopy.

Last night was very sad for Brian. Because of Eve's exposure to chicken pox virus, it was the last day she could come to the hospital. Both of them cried when it was time to go home. As much as we all (OK, at least the adults) know it's not forever, it sure felt like it. And of course, in the back of my mind, I feared it might be.

This afternoon, however, Brian was unexpectedly permitted to go outside for 20 minutes with Eve in the vicinity. He was out there, slathered in sunscreen, wearing a gown and gloves and his "Indiana Jones" hat. Eve was supposed to stay 10 feet away from him due to the whole Shingles Extravaganza.

Now, you might think this would be emotionally difficult — Eve wanting her Daddy, Daddy wanting to hold her, separated by force, Eve kicking and screaming.
You don't know our kid too well.

Eve thought this was the greatest game in the world: Chase Daddy. She chased him and he ran and she laughed and chased some more, etc. It was so funny to see Indiana c.Diff running away from a one-year-old. It really cheered everyone up.

Meanwhile, the family medicine folks now are thinking that perhaps Joe doesn't have shingles after all. They're thinking now maybe it's a staph infection. If so, it's very treatable and Joe can come see Brian tomorrow. However, that would mean that Eve got her varicella vaccine for no reason, causing a most unnecessary and really annoying exile from Daddy, not to mention great undo stress on Mommy. The docs finally cultured Joe's skin yesterday (why couldn't they do that in the first place?) so maybe we'll have an actual answer tomorrow.

Joe is now allowed to care for Eve, so they're hanging out this morning. Brian is really tired and so am I. He's been in the hospital almost four weeks and that's just a really long time. We are hoping against hope that tomorrow's endoscopy will give us some answers or at least a plan to get him home.

Meanwhile, about seven trillion people a day come into his room and say, "Are you still here? Why are you here? You're too healthy to be here! You must like it here." This is funny only about the first ten times, after which we plot violence.

In case you were wondering, Brian Wants To Go Home!!!. He looks good, he feels pretty good, and the next person who implies that somehow he's in the hospital of his own free will answers to me.

naomi

Date: Mon, 14 Jun 1999
Subject: Day +23: Brian on drugs

Disclaimer: Brian has threatened to divorce me for including some of the things that are in this update, so I may be back in Pittsburgh sooner than you thought!

First, a follow up on yesterday. Brian received a phone call last night from Steve Cohen, his former next door neighbor. Steve had not seen Brian in outpatient and so figured, correctly, that Brian was stuck inpatient and that his spirits could use a boost. Brian was so incredibly touched by this gesture from someone who had so much else going on in his life. It was really nice.

I went up to the hospital as usual this morning but, unlike usual, didn't go ask for his counts at 9 sharp. The floor staff makes unmerciful fun of me because I'm always there at exactly 9 AM, while his counts are never there at exactly 9 AM. Look, I care about his health, OK?
At around 9:20, the nurse stuck her head in and asked if we wanted his counts. "I don't know," I replied, "Do we?" Well, the answer was a resounding yes. Everything was way up. My husband the marrow stud! About time!

Transport came to get Brian for his endoscopy around 12:45. They brought this gurney to transport him on, which Brian absolutely refused to ride on. So he walked in front of the gurney, wearing his gown and gloves, all the way to gastroenterology.

I was allowed to view Brian's endoscopy, which, from a nerdly point of view, was kind of cool. My biggest problem with it, actually, was that it made me motion sick. They thread a camera down his throat into his stomach and upper small intestine, and it makes the Omnimax theater look like a grainy beta-max video. I wasn't terribly grossed out because I just didn't know enough about what I was seeing. The only thing that bothered me to watch was the actual taking of biopsy samples.

Anyway, what they saw was consistent with some mild gut GVH, but could possibly be other things, like perhaps a small ulcer or just some irritation from throwing up. We will get the result of the biopsies tomorrow and then they can make some decisions about how best to treat him.

The greatest part of this experience, however, was the drugs. They put Brian on Versed® and fentanyl. First of all, he just refused to be sedated. He was lying on the bed, a mouth guard in his mouth, enough drugs to kill a moose in his blood stream, and the docs kept saying, "You awake Brian?" Now, a simple "yes" would have sufficed. But Brian was stoned, mind you, so he kept trying to expound at great length on his state of consciousness. Except no one could understand him because the guard was in his mouth. So they just kept saying, "OK, Brian, close your eyes," and they would give him more, and try again. As they were about to start the procedure, Brian demanded a pillow for his back. Ornery guy I married.

After they were done and he was starting to come out of sedation, we had a conversation that went something like this:

B: Did you see cool stuff?
N: Kind of. It made me motion sick.
B: (laughing) What did they find?
N: (Brief synopsis of what they saw)
B: Oh. How long are you staying?
N: I'll stay until you go back to your room.
B: What's this stupid pillow doing on my back?
(long pause)
B: Was it cool?
N: Yes, dear.
B: What did they find?
N: (Brief synopsis)
B: Oh. Are you going home?
N: I'm staying until you go back to your room.
B: Thanks. I had a great dream last night. (Lecherous look appears in his eye)
N: Tell me about it later.
B: Are you going home now?
N: After you're in your room.
B: What did they find?

You see how this goes. Anyway, things do seem to be headed in the right direction, at least for now. More tomorrow, as you know!

naomi

Lucky for me, not only does Brian not remember any of the embarrassing stuff I reported in yesterday's e-mail, but he doesn't remember threatening me to keep me from reporting it. Phew.

Brian's counts this morning were back to their weird selves. Platelets were up, hematocrit stable, whites down and ANC way down. At rounds, I asked Dr. W., "What's up with his counts?" He sagely replied, "They're going up and down a lot." Years of specialized medical training, folks! He reiterated very firmly that Brian's strong platelet counts are very unusual for a MUD recipient at this stage and that they indicate that the graft has taken hold. He said, "I don't mean to belittle it, but I'm really, really, really not worried about it." For once, that was good enough for me.

The first really good news of the day is that Brian's second culture for c.Diff was negative, so he is out of isolation. I felt positively naked sitting in his room in shorts and a t-shirt, no gown, no gloves. What a thrill.
The second news, which is, on balance, good, is that they did find mild GVHD in his gut. It is sufficiently mild that it would not require treatment were it not for his inability to keep that pesky cyclosporine down.

We met with Dr. W. for quite some time this afternoon and discussed options. Brian decided to participate in a study of beclomethasone, a steroid which they give topically (i.e. you swallow it). It's not systemic and so doesn't have all the nasty side effects of prednisone, which is the steroid patients with GVHD usually take. The bad part is that beclomethasone works more slowly and, of course, it doesn't work for everyone.
Presuming Brian can keep the bec down, Dr. W. is willing to let him go home after six doses. He will still be getting cyclosporine and itraconazole IV, so he'll be at the clinic the vast majority of the time during the day. But Brian would rather do it outpatient and be allowed to go home when he's done. I second that emotion.

So, if all goes well, he will go home sometime on Thursday. If all does not go well, he'll upchuck the bec tonight, start prednisone, and still go home at the end of the week. Unless things go really badly, in which case he'll develop some brand new problem. This will not happen. I refuse.

naomi

So far, so good.

Brian yacked up his first dose of bec last night but has kept down the subsequent three. Brian's counts today are downright macho. His platelet count is 99. 99! Can you believe it? That is 11 times what it was two weeks ago! That is 2/3 of normal! That is a number we never expected to see again.

No firm word on going home as yet, and we wouldn't believe them if they gave us firm word anyway. We've been burned too many times. But, in an act of sheer optimism, I washed the quilt on our bed at home. I'm actually starting to believe, if only just a little. I've allowed myself a few moments of faith that I might be married to this guy for a little bit longer. Brian's mood is much better, too. Things are looking up.

Today was my day to sleep in, because I wasn't coming to the hospital until the afternoon. Unfortunately, this was also Eve's day to wake up really early. So much for that. You know you're in trouble when you have to beg your spouse, who is less than a month out from a bone marrow transplant, to walk fewer laps because you are too tired to keep up.

We received a package from my brother and sister-in-law today containing a birthday present for Eve and presents for both Brian and me. His was a bug gun. It's a toy catapult gun that shoots rubber bugs. The accompanying note said it was for him to shoot at people who "bug" him about why he's still in the hospital. There was also an accompanying picture drawn by my niece, apparently of him slamming his door in said people's faces. I like her style.

My gift hearkened back to Brian's second day of conditioning when I wrote in my update about Michael, the little boy with the great toys. I wrote that I admired his coloring set. Well, Abe and Colleen and the kids sent me a set with about 20 million colors of markers, pastels, crayons, colored pencils, and paints, with a sketch pad to go with. Now, if only I had any artistic talent to speak of . . .

On a more serious note, I've become kind of friendly with the husband of a woman on my floor. He shows me pictures of his grandkids, I show him pictures of Eve, we ask after each other's spouses. Jenny, his wife, has been going downhill for about a week but he's been very upbeat. Then, a couple of days ago, she went into ICU. When I saw him today and asked how she was, he said, very matter-of-factly, "I think we're going to lose her." In the odd way that hospital contacts often are, I realized as I talked to him about it that I didn't even know his name. I was amazed he could manage a laugh when I asked him.

However annoyed and sad we may be that Brian is still in the hospital, in our hearts we now know he's coming home someday. Others are not so for-tunate. My heart just aches for Chip (that's his name), and I am so frustrated that I can't do more than offer a kind word. It is, of course, the families where the patient is not doing as well who are around more, and so we get to know them more. When things get better, the whole floor celebrates. When things look bad, you realize what a blessing it is to have your family intact for one more day.

I hope to bring word of a miracle for Jenny and a homecoming for Brian tomorrow. We pray for both and bank on neither.

naomi

Date: Thu, 17 Jun 1999
Subject: Day +26: One day more

If all goes well, by this time tomorrow Brian will be home. There are no more hurdles to cross to get him here; he just has to not get worse. Eve will have to stay a safe distance away until around the 28th, but at night Brian and I will be kicking each other in bed, which will be a pleasure.

Several people have pointed out that between Eve and adjusting Brian's hydration at night, I won't be getting much sleep. I suggested that I make Brian's pump "beep it out" until it learns not to go off at night. What do you think? Makes about as much sense to me as making Eve "cry it out," but then, that's me.

The news from Brian's floor is mixed. When I arrived this morning, I found that Jenny, the woman I wrote about yesterday, was out of ICU! Chip simply said, "She's back!" Apparently she woke up last night and is breathing easier. She's certainly not out of the woods but, as Chip put it, "I didn't expect we'd be here this morning."

Other news is not as good. As Brian and I were out for his morning walk, we heard a beeping we hadn't heard before over the call system, and the nurses started running from everywhere — a code. As we hurried back to Brian's room to get out of the way, we saw where everyone was going: Pedro's room. Pretty soon we heard the sobs and saw his wife walking through the hall with Moreen.

Pedro died this morning. I don't know whether his family at all expected this, but we certainly didn't expect it. Pedro's family is Spanish-speaking and so, due to the language barrier, we didn't really get to know them the way we have some others. But we always shared a smile and a nod when we walked laps together. Pedro had a son a few months younger than Eve, and they've made faces at each other a few times.

It's interesting, there are two sounds you know occur on BMT halls and yet rarely hear, and they are very disturbing. One is the sound of someone throwing up, and the other is the sound of sobbing. There was a lot of the latter this morning on the hall. Actually, come to think of it, I heard the former too. I saw Pedro's brother in the hall, but I didn't know how to offer comfort even if I did speak the same language. This is what we all fear going into this process, and it makes us aware that Brian is still here by the grace of God.

We are very blessed that Brian is doing so well. I think his doctors are glad that he's leaving, because we are getting a tad too punchy with them. When Dr. W. came in to examine Brian yesterday, the nurse was shouting, "Shoot him with the bug gun!"

naomi

Chapter 6:
Elvis Has Left the Building

Date: Fri, 18 Jun 1999
Subject: Day +27: Elvis has left the building!

Yes, folks, you heard that right! Brian left the hospital today around 12:30. He of course insisted on walking home, so Mark and two of Mark's coworkers loaded all the stuff into the car and then we walked home, sending Joe up the hill to get the car after we got back.

Brian still must report to the outpatient clinic twice a day for two hours to get his cyclosporine IV and his itraconazole IV. He also has assorted appointments. But he is living at home! Brian's departure from the BMT ward was an emotional affair. One of the nurses cried, his Fellow gave him a big hug, and we made tentative plans to take our kids to the park together sometime. Brian really made some friends on the staff in his month in the hospital.

This afternoon, Brian, Eve and I went to a hat store where I bought Brian a really snazzy hat for Father's Day. He has to wear hats all the time when outdoors, so I thought we'd really do it up. It's a Stetson, Panama style, with an upturned rear brim. Frankly, he looks like he might be trying to sell you something. Very sharp.

This evening, Brian cooked salmon for dinner. It was by far the best meal I've had since he's been in. What have I been eating? I can't remember. I set up his pump to start his hydration and then he went up to the clinic for his evening cyclosporine.
While he's gone, in addition to writing this, I had to give Eve a bath, put her to bed, do the dishes, draw flushes for his Hickman line, get his other bag of hydration ready to go and change the sheets on the bed. And you know what, I don't really care because he's home!

Well, gotta go burp some IV bags. More tomorrow!

naomi

Mark has now dubbed Brian "the blood stud." His platelet count today was the highest it has been on any blood test that was ever reported to Brian in his life.

This morning, we got up bright and early and went to clinic for Brian's AM cyclosporine and itraconazole and for his "new discharge clinic" appointment. Since it's a weekend, he didn't meet the doctors who will be caring for him on an ongoing basis, but rather the people who drew the short straw and were on this weekend.

The nurse and the doctor talked with us about how he was feeling (pretty good) and any symptoms he was having (not really). They confirmed that he is the only patient either of them has ever met who went through the whole transplant without ever needing TPN to supplement food. I find this really poetic since his gut is his one and only complication. Basically, they flipped through his chart and remarked repeatedly on how good he looked and how well he's doing, and then the appointment was over. I sat there and grinned like an idiot through the whole thing. He's home!

On Monday, he will meet with his regular doctors and the nutritionist. It's harder for him to eat in the real world than it was in the hospital if only because the menu isn't as extensive and someone actually has to make it — usually him because he never lets me cook.

After clinic, I came home, played with Eve and put her down for a nap. Then I did something unheard of. I slept. For an hour and a half. I feel like a wild woman.

This afternoon, Brian, Eve and I went for a walk and took Eve to the park. The highlight of this was when a bird decided to do its business on my shoulder. Which, when the person you are walking with is supposed to stay away from animal droppings, can be somewhat tricky to clean up. Ick.

This evening, Brian had dinner with his parents while I took Mark and Eve out for a nice dinner. We all earned it this last month, and Brian heartily encouraged us to go party it up.

Tomorrow is Father's Day, and we are thrilled that Daddy gets to spend it with his kid.

naomi

Today was downright dull. Brian's only clinic appointments were for his IV meds, and the rest of the day was spent lolling around, napping (for him), watching tube (for me), etc. Eve gave him a little card that said, "Dad, the reasons I love you are more than the stars in the sky. More than the grains of sand on the beach. More than the hairs on your head." And then on the inside it said, "OK, maybe that last one isn't such a good comparison." She even signed it "by self."

Brian is starting to get into the swing of outpatient life. By swing, we mean "Pattern of remembering to take meds, not puking them up and scheduling hydration." A lot of caregivers count out meds, work the pump and change the Hickman dressing for the patient, but Brian prefers to do all that himself. This makes me feel pretty extraneous, but it's important for him to feel like he can take care of himself.

In the middle of last night, when his IV hydration was done and the pump beeped, he was so tired he absolutely could not figure out why it was beeping and what he was supposed to do about it. But of course, I'm not allowed to just climb over him in bed and press "off" because that would be taking over his responsibility. So I had to watch him fumble to the bathroom, dragging the knapsack with his pump behind him, and listen to it beep behind the door for five minutes before he woke up enough to figure out that he needed to turn it off and flush his line. He is so used to sleeping through this sort of thing because, in the hospital, a beeping pump is the nurse's responsibility. This really is taking some getting used to.

Another interesting issue is keeping track of his food. Although he no longer has to have all input and output measured (ah, the joys of flushing your own toilet!), he has to keep a detailed record of all food and drink, including precise amounts of everything. Tonight for dinner, his mom and I cooked up a Chinese feast. Brian sat at the table with a pad and paper and tried to keep track of what he was eating, which was pretty funny, because he eats a lot: 7 chicken potstickers, 2 tbs. sweet and sour sauce, one cup rice, 1/4 lb. chicken, stir fried with 3/4 cups vegetables, 1 cup blueberries (at $4.00 a box, nothing's too good for my sweetie!), 3 spoonfuls Breyer's mint chip ice cream, 2 Almond Roca, 24 oz iced tea. Can you believe that his gut is his problem?

Today felt positively empty because it was the first time in over a month they haven't gotten his blood counts. A weird, paranoid piece of me fears that, in fact, all his counts dropped to zero yesterday, and nobody will know until tomorrow, and by then it will be too late! AGGGGH!

Oh, and my big accomplishment for the day is that I took half an hour and mucked around with the art set my brother's family sent. Great fun. I never had much of a knack for it, but if given free reign I really enjoy drawing and painting. I even managed to sketch our living room in Pittsburgh in such a way that Brian recognized it (no kidding, he really did!). It also helps that, when I do relaxation exercises lately, I find myself visualizing our Pittsburgh house as a "safe place," so it's very much in my mind. Who ever thought I'd be homesick for that lovely pink carpeting? Don't blame me, it's a rental!

naomi

Date: Mon, 21 Jun 1999
Subject: Day +30

Like all good outpatient days, today began with Brian calling from the clinic to tell me to get my tail up there because, without telling him, they had moved his clinic appointment to 9 from 1:30. I called Barb, she came over, I raced up the hill, arriving at 9:02, and . . . nobody showed up for 20 minutes for the appointment. Could have predicted that, couldn't you?

When folks did show, we met with the nurse, the physician's assistant and the attending. I can summarize their reaction to Brian in one word — stupor. I swear, they just kept staring at him. At one point, the nurse actually said, "Are you sure we gave you chemo?" He is just doing amazingly well.

The hurdle that remains is getting his meds down orally. He agreed to cut back some on his Ativan® in the next day or two and see how he felt and then go from there. They gave us a definite impression that they don't see him staying here the whole 100 days, although that can change in an instant, and they made that clear too.

It was sort of old home week at the clinic. Jack Sarfaty stopped by the infusion room to share high fives with Brian on his release. We also saw Steve and Sharon Cohen. Steve shared his secret for getting down his morning cyclosporine — rugelach. Rugelach is a Jewish pastry. Cinnamon rugelach before your cyclosporine dose apparently does the trick. I suggested that Steve write the "Jewish Man's Guide to BMT" and include this tip. It was great to feel like so many people were glad to see Brian out. We certainly are!

In the afternoon, we met with the nutritionist, who used the word "amazed" repeatedly to refer to Brian's eating and drinking. He apparently managed close to 4000 calories yesterday, which alarms me because I'm eating right along with him. Luckily, we don't have a bathroom scale out here, because I doubt that at 4000 calories a day my weight is anywhere near stable. Drinking Caramel Frappucinos to combat stress probably doesn't help much.

Back home, I think Brian and I are both discovering that having him home isn't the be all and end all of happiness. I'm still super-tired and he is finding the number of things he's supposed to remember to do very annoying. Getting out the door in the morning is a major task, what with showering, sunscreen, various skin creams, changing his Hickman dressing, meds, flushes, and on and on. I could probably help alleviate some of that, but he won't let me. He needs a nap every afternoon, and between clinic time for his meds, naps, and trying to stay at arms distance from Eve, we still aren't seeing all that much of one another. But still, it's better than being in. And everyone's "stupor" reminds us that he is doing amazingly way better than most, and that's wonderful.

Brian's platelets are up today (so much for my "down to 0" paranoia)

121

and everything else is nice and steady. They are only going to see him in clinic once a week plus twice weekly blood draws. It is a little unnerving to go from them measuring and checking everything 14 billion times a day to "see you next week." It feels like we're walking the high wire without a net.

If you'll excuse me, I have to go try on the sequined tutu that goes with this circus act.

naomi

Date: Tue, 22 Jun 1999
Subject: Day +31

Today, Brian had his day 28 bone marrow aspiration.

This marrow was to check two things:
1) How much of the marrow is donor cells and 2) Does it look healthy?

The answers we're hoping for here are
1) over 90% and 2) yes.

We don't have any reason to expect otherwise, but you never know. Brian had a relatively easy time of it, thanks to the fentanyl, and came home and hung out, did laundry and generally had a relaxing afternoon. Believe it or not, Brian has no clinic appointments scheduled until next week. So I may not bother to write every day from here on in, because there won't, we hope, be much to say.

I'm finding it really hard to convey the balance we feel like there is in this situation. On the one hand, Brian is doing really well, and we're very thankful for that. On the other hand, our starting point — a bone marrow transplant — is inherently lousy. I think it's hard for friends to talk to us and be supportive without pitying us.

One person called to tell me about a big health problem her husband was having, and then followed it up with, "But your life is much worse than mine." And while, if I take a deep breath, I know she meant well, that really didn't help. On the other hand, some people go to the opposite extreme, presuming that if our lives are not a big tragedy that we really don't need anything from them. Because I'm a tad paranoid, I wind up feeling like everyone says, "Oh, thank God, that's over. Now we can go back to ignoring her." I know my friends have good intentions. I just don't know how to tell them what I need and keep my dignity at the same time.

We're looking forward to some days of doin' nothin' coming up, and when we get back to doin' somethin', we'll let you know.

naomi

Date: Thu, 24 Jun 1999
Subject: Day +33

Today, Brian's nausea was somewhat better but he developed some diarrhea. And you know what the answer to diarrhea (and everything else) is — "let's culture that." That's not so bad when you're inpatient. They do it and you don't know about it. But outpatient it requires actually creating this sample for them. I won't go into the details, but yuck. Luckily, when I say that Brian insists on doing everything for himself, that includes everything.

Brian is still unwilling to try his cyclosporine orally, so we're on for another weekend of trips to the infusion room. I suspect that, if he hasn't tried it by Monday, the doctors will start noodging him a little more. At this point, his inability to try is probably more psychosomatic than anything else. However, the last time I said that it turned out he had GVHD of the gut, so who knows?

The good news continues to be his counts, particularly his platelets. One of the nurses threatened to make him go to the blood bank to donate platelets! He has twice as many platelets now as he has in the last 14 years. I know for a fact that I have myself donated platelets with a count lower than his. It's just so amazing, after all these years of saying he's fine except for his platelets, that they should come in so strongly.

I am writing this on my last 20 minutes of "shore leave." My in-laws took Eve for 5 hours this afternoon so Brian and I could do fascinating things like clean the closet. I went to have my hair done, and we went up to the BMT ward, brought the staff an ice cream cake and took pictures of some of our favorite nurses.

As nice as it was to "return in triumph" to the floor, we were saddened to see that two of Brian's neighbors had passed away since he checked off the floor 6 days ago. One was Jenny, the woman whose husband I wrote about last week. This really seemed to pull Brian up short — to realize how easily that could have been him and how lucky he has been thus far.

The only way I can reach Chip is by giving a letter to the social worker, who will then forward it along. What can I say to someone who is living my worst fear?

This morning I had coffee with Caryn, whose husband, Richard, is on day 84 of a transplant here. Her husband and Brian are both doing really well, but Caryn and I are both showing signs of wear. We were both pretty pooped this morning. It was nice to spend time with someone who knows that, even when things are great for a BMT patient, they are pretty yucky from any normal point of view.

naomi

Date: Fri, 25 Jun 1999
Subject: Day +34: The 8 buck a month Ativan® habit

Today, Brian and I went for a talk with the Pain and Toxicity specialist because Brian's been having some trouble getting off of Ativan®. I guess I should explain exactly what happened.

Ativan® is an anti-anxiety medication that is commonly used to treat nausea. After much experimentation while in the hospital, Brian felt it was the only one that didn't knock him out and he didn't have a nasty reaction to. In the hospital, he got Ativan® IV with some frequency. When he left the hospital, he took oral Ativan® an hour before his beclomethasone dose. He didn't wait to get nauseous. He just took it to "stay ahead" of the nausea.

On Monday, the doctors suggested he switch to half mg doses instead of 1mg. He felt pretty good, and so pretty much stopped taking the Ativan® altogether by Tuesday.

Monday night, I had a less-than-lucid conversation with him in the middle of the night. He couldn't sleep and kept using the words "chemical dependency," which seemed rather apt. He was half asleep but clearly very agitated. In the morning, he was totally frenetic and cleaned the house, which I didn't mind.

Tuesday night, he was absolutely frantic. He couldn't sleep, his mind was racing, he wouldn't stay in bed. He finally took half a mg of Ativan® and got a few hours of sleep, but was totally exhausted on Wednesday. When he came home from infusion on Wednesday, he went to take a nap, but couldn't. He described it as, "if a dream is a TV show, I'm watching the news, and it's a new show every 30 seconds." This didn't make a whole lot of sense to me, honestly, but it was pretty scary to see. His doc told him to start the Ativan® again, at least in small doses, and made an appointment with Pain and Tox for him.

The Pain and Tox doctor's reaction to this, after hearing both Brian's description and mine (which weren't exactly the same), was, "Sounds ghastly." He said that, although Ativan® is of a class of drugs that people can have trouble with, Brian is the first person he's run across who had this much trouble getting off it. He gave us a little lecture about what causes addiction and particularly what causes it in this particular drug, and then gave Brian something of a schedule for coming off the Ativan® slowly.

Brian complained that no one had warned him about this, but, to be fair, he hadn't done what the docs told him to do, which was go to half mg doses. He had just stopped. The doctor said that although they might have warned him, since this almost never happens it isn't something they think to tell you about.

I know this description sounds pretty awful, but frankly it hasn't been that bad. The house is nice and clean, for one. And, while Brian is pretty tired from all this and pretty shaken by the notion that he actually has a "drug problem," it's such a minor drug problem that it's hard to take it too seriously. Besides this, life is pretty boring here. Eve is asleep, and I'm headed that way.

Good night and good luck to all!

naomi

Date: Mon, 28 Jun 1999
Subject: Day +37

This morning, Brian woke up, put his little tootsies on the floor, stood up, and suddenly had an urge to pee so strong he almost didn't make it to the bathroom. Over the next three hours, he estimates that he peed 1.5 liters. He also had a dull ache in his bladder, felt rotten in his stomach, and had lost some serious weight (about four and a half pounds in the last few days).

Luckily, however, today was clinic day, so when he went for his infusion they just had him pee in a cup and told him to talk to the doctors at his appointment this afternoon.

Meanwhile, at home, our building management had been kind enough to inform us there would be no water from 9 AM to 5 PM. This would be a minor inconvenience for most folks, but for a BMT patient, no water means no hand washing, no flushing and no washing fruits and vegetables. This rendered the apartment uninhabitable. So we camped out at Joe's for the day, where Eve steadfastly refused to nap anywhere other than on Joe's shoulder. Cute, yes. Practical, no.

Brian and I went up to clinic for his nutrition and clinic appointments in the afternoon. Apparently BMT patients retain a ton of water during transplant, so it's not unusual to lose a fair amount of water weight at this stage. The nutritionist was unconcerned about the weight loss.

The clinic appointment brought some good news. Brian's day 28 marrow showed normal cell growth (no MDS) but hypocellular marrow, meaning that he doesn't have as many marrow cells as a normal person. That's not really surprising if you think about it. His has only been there for 31 days! His marrow was normal for this stage of transplant, however.

Brian's marrow has 95% donor cells. This of course upset me. The overachiever in me wants to get 100% every time. However, his doctor explained that there is no clinical difference between 95% and 100%. She said that, in fact, if I were to have a marrow done, they could very well find 1-5% cells that aren't me in my marrow, and we know that's wrong. The test just isn't that sensitive. Also, if Brian does have residual old cells, his GVHD may well kill them off.

I'll be honest and admit that I was not totally satisfied with this explanation. It's all well and good to say there's no difference between 95% and 100%. But the fact of the matter is that other patients have 100% on their tests. The notion that there is any of Brian's old marrow in there at all makes me nervous, and I then, of course, have to be mad at the doctor for being so stupid and not realizing there is a crisis at hand!!

Brian agreed to try to take his cyclosporine orally starting tomorrow. He is very nervous about this and trying hard not to psych himself out, but it is difficult. We'll see how it goes. Their take on the pee factor was that he may have some type of urinary tract infection, most likely viral.

After clinic, I went to the hospital to visit with Cyndi Prichard, a BMT-talk person whose husband, Don, is on day 12 of a transplant. She had told me his room number on the 11th floor, but the room was vacant when I got there, which made me very scared. As it turned out, they had moved Don down to the 9th floor and into ICU. Don is experiencing hyper-acute GVH, a very, very serious side effect, and he is on all sorts of aggressive and experimental treatments. Cyndi is living at the hospital with him. I have to say that Cyndi seemed very put together under the circumstances. She did mention, however, that she can't stand being told that she's doing fine when it doesn't feel that way, so I'm obligated to tell you she looked like heck.

While on the 9th floor, I was pleased to see that two of Brian's neighbors who were transplanted within a week or so of him were moving out today. It was great to have some positive news for a change.

Brian's nutritionist is now actually encouraging him carefully to go out to eat, since that is something he really enjoys. We are hoping that this week, when a friend is visiting from home, we can go to Benihana, which is one of those places where they throw your food around and cook it right in front of you. We thought that was a good choice, since you certainly know the food hasn't been sitting out since it was cooked! Brian is really looking forward to this.

Well, off to bed for me. I remember sleep very fondly.

naomi

Date: Tue, 29 Jun 1999
Subject: Day +38: Who are these people and what have they done with my family?

Today marked two majorly historic moments in the Summer of Marrow at the Zikmund-Fishers.

First, Brian has now taken two oral doses of cyclosporine, kept it down, and lived to tell about it. I wouldn't say he's happy about it, mind you, but it's a step, and perhaps it will get easier.

Second, Ms. Eve, a.k.a. the sleepless wonder, went to sleep around 9:30 PM and woke up for the first time around 5:30 AM. It was light when she went down and light when she got up, so we're counting it. It only took her nearly 13 months to sleep through the night for the first time. I, of course, didn't sleep through the night because, when she didn't wake up, I became convinced that something horrible had occurred but didn't want to go check on her because then I might wake her up. We're trying not to get used to it, because it will certainly change.

Today was a boring day. Boring is good! No doctor's appointments or anything, just hanging out, doing laundry, etc. This evening, we went with Mark to our favorite ice cream place on the lake. This place specializes in mixing stuff into your ice cream, but Brian was wary of the cleanliness of the mixing surface, so he had them plop his ice cream directly into a bowl and pour the stuff on top. Good enough! He was very forward about telling them why he needed this, and they were totally unfazed.

After we got our ice cream, we went to the park across the street so Eve could run around. We're sitting there at a picnic table, when Eve makes the tell-tale "grunt and turn red" faces indicating that finding a changing station might be advantageous to all concerned. As we're discussing where one might be, all of a sudden a squirrel jumps on the table and starts going after Mark's ice cream. So he jumps up and Brian starts trying to chase this fearless beast away, but Eve has no sense and is trying to touch it.

We decide that, if we can't get the squirrel to leave, we'll leave, so I scoop Eve up and we walk away. And the squirrel starts chasing us. Fast. We start walking faster. Finally, Brian takes the stroller and chases the squirrel into a tree, saying, "I'm bigger than you!" But the squirrel starts chasing us again. We must have been quite a sight: bald guy pushing empty stroller, short woman carrying poopy baby, guy carrying everyone's ice cream, being chased by Killer Squirrel from Hell.

All in all, not a bad day. Life is feeling fairly normal around here, or at least as normal as things can be when you have as many doctor's appointments as Brian does and a tube hanging out of your chest.

naomi

The last several days have been medically uneventful. Brian's counts are continuing to be strong. In fact, I don't actually have them committed to memory anymore. I never thought that day would come. His platelets are dropping but still in the normal range, so no one is concerned.

On Wednesday, our friend Nancy from Pittsburgh arrived with her parents. Brian had his debut performance at eating out — we went to Benihana. We went just as they were opening for dinner and Brian had to be pretty careful. He washed his hands after ordering and skipped the salad and sprouts. Salad is OK if everything is washed within an inch of its life, but in a restaurant that's unlikely. Sprouts are not OK period. We had a nice time and stuffed our faces, but Brian said he still felt like there are many reminders that things aren't normal. I felt it too. It's amazing how aware you become of how poorly people handle food sometimes. The chef putting raw meat onto the grill with his fork and spatula and then using the same utensils to serve vegetables particularly disturbed me.

Nancy brought us wonderful presents. For me, warm fleece socks for this cold summer, a coffee mug and candy rum balls. For Eve, three Sandra Boynton board books. For Brian, a copy of *Alexander and the Terrible, Horrible, No Good, Very Bad Day*, a favorite of ours and very appropriate given the national origin of his donor. As the book keeps telling us, "some days are like that, even in Australia". The Aussie jokes are coming fast and furious, but the award still goes to our friend Betsy, who sent Brian vegemite. Yuck.

Today, Brian took Eve by himself twice — once while I went up to talk to our social worker and once when I went to give blood (hint, hint, noodge. There's a shortage, folks. No one else is going to do this for you!). He can do just about everything baby-care-wise except nurse her, which was never exactly a strong suit in the first place, and change her diapers. Sure enough, she pooped while I was giving blood and I had a mess to clean up when I got home, but I think he really appreciated having the time to reconnect with her. She's changed a lot in the last six weeks and he feels sometimes like he doesn't know her patterns anymore. Luckily, she's a pretty forgiving kid and she thinks he's a major celebrity, so they pretty much have a love-fest when they're together.

My appointment with Moreen was really important. Truth told, things haven't been going that well between Brian and me. I actually walked into her office and announced I was going back to Pittsburgh. "No, you're not," she replied. "Yes, I am," I said. And on it went. She assured me that a lot of couples find this stage of transplant particularly difficult. She said that, as long as I didn't actually get on the plane, I was within the range of normal.

I've been doing the "I am woman hear me roar" independence thing for a month and it's hard to make space for Brian to come back. He's in my way, and I feel like allowing him to do anything takes away from the independence I've established without him. I resent any implication that I can't do things myself, and I take just about everything as an implication that I can't do things myself.

On the other hand, there's a difficult balance between the fact that he feels well, all things considered, and the fact that in any real sense he's still kinda sick. It's hard to know how much he really needs from me and how much I'm entitled to a break. I mean, unlike most caregivers, I never rig up his pump or flush his line or help with meds, so what do I need a break from? But I do need one, and I feel guilty about it. And I get mad at him, because I feel like he's doing well whenever anyone on the outside asks, but as soon as I want him to do something around the house he's too sick. But then, if he does do it, he's taking away from my independence. Neither of us can win.

Moreen also pointed out that Brian and I seem to be at our best when we have a joint project to undertake. Most of our marriage — most of our relationship, even — has been one joint project after another. First, we were trying to get through college. After graduation, we were finding an apartment and setting up a life together in New York. Then we were planning the wedding. Then we were moving to Pittsburgh. Then we were trying to get pregnant and dealing with the pain of infertility and the Herculean task which was managing our fertility care. Then we were having a baby. Then we were getting ready for Brian's transplant. But now what? What if we find out that, when things are pretty even and steady, we don't actually like each other very much? Moreen suggested we try to find a new joint project, but pointed out it didn't need to be a crisis.

Brian and I spent much of the evening having a serious conversation about all of this, just trying to get feelings into the open. Even though the transplant has been amazingly trouble free, this situation is really stressful. We're on each other's nerves, and we needed to admit it. I don't know what our next joint project will be, but we're working on it. And, at least for now, I'm not getting on the plane.

Eve spent much of this evening demanding that we read certain pages of *Mr. Brown Can Moo, Can You?* over and over and over and over. And she can find these pages herself. And make the noises. Have you ever heard a 13-month-old baby do a hippopotamus chewing gum? It's pretty funny. Eve is so smart she even knows how to hang up the phone while nursing. Today, she hung up on my mother. Which would be funny were my parents not calling from Italy. Oops.

The excitement of the night came around 6:45 PM when the building started to shake. I noticed it immediately. It took Brian, desensitized from years of living in California, somewhat longer. It was a 5.6 earthquake. Not the biggest in the world, but big enough to make you stop and wonder whether it was going to be bigger. Very exciting.

Date: Tue, 6 Jul 1999
Subject: Day +45 (long and somewhat off-topic)

Once again, there isn't a whole lot medically to report. Here's the bullet.

Brian's counts are stable, his mood is pretty good and they took him off hydration today. His only major issue at the moment (and it is a very minor major issue) is a case of folliculitis seemingly caused by his hats and some sweat, which has caused his forehead to break out in zit-like spots. It's so minor they're not treating it. They just want him to take off his hat when indoors and wash his head more. Remember, before transplant they were calling him "folliculitis guy?" They were right! He remains on IV itra for another week, mostly because he doesn't want to switch to the icky oral liquid junk, and that's just about it.

We had a really nice weekend. Saturday afternoon, while Eve napped, Mark and I broke out my art set and did some drawing. I came up with a kind of impressionistic view of the mountains as seen from Brian's first hospital room. I'm finding drawing places and views from particular moments in time very therapeutic. I could wax poetic about why that is but I'm not sure it would make any sense. Thus far I've done passable sketches of our house in Pittsburgh and the chapel at my high school. I find the mere fact that these places are as etched in my mind as they must be to draw them fairly well gives me a much-needed feeling of groundedness in a very ungrounded situation.

I'm also finding being out here somewhat freeing in an odd way. I feel like, "I'm thousands of miles from home, I don't know anyone, what do I have to lose, I might as well be someone else!" The mere fact that I've taken up drawing at all is part of that. As a second part, on Saturday night I colored my hair. Now, I want to make two things abundantly clear. First is that my purpose in coloring my hair was not to cover my ever-expanding gray. I rather like my gray, thank you. Second is that I used a temporary hair color which supposedly washes out in 24 shampoos. But I did, indeed, for the very first time in my tiny life, use hair coloring — a "bright burgundy." Reviews are mixed. It actually doesn't look very different unless you are extremely well acquainted with my hair. But just doing it felt good. If Brian can have a snazzy new summer do, then so can I!!!

On Sunday, I went to the hospital to see Cyndi, my Internet buddy whose husband, Don, is inpatient. Don is having a lot of problems with his lungs and the docs are scrambling to find an assortment of treatments for him. At the moment he is taking an experimental treatment for hyper-acute GVHD as well as mega-doses of steroids for radiation-induced pneumonia. The situation is pretty severe.

I brought Cyndi a care package for every mood — a squirt bottle, a foam baseball bat, some body wash, and some candy. The candy was a big hit. You can see why Cyndi and I get along. I stopped by to see her again

133

today and she mentioned that she was getting in trouble for using the squirt bottle on the medical staff. Good for her!

For Independence Day, Mark managed to convince us that Chinese food was traditional, so Brian whipped up a feast. As he was cooking part one of this feast, I had my back to him and heard a "whoosh" sound and the kitchen suddenly got, um, brighter. Then I heard Brian, in his wonderful, understated way, say, "Um . . ." I turned around to see a rather large grease fire in the wok.

Now, not being a good cook has its drawbacks. But it also has the advantage that I know how to put out a grease fire from personal experience. So I grabbed the baking soda out of the fridge and a major crisis was averted, although the apartment was relatively smoky for a while.

The rest of the meal (three courses plus dessert) went off without a hitch, and we stuffed ourselves until we couldn't move. Our plan for the fireworks was simple: since there are two major fireworks shows over two different bodies of water, and since both of these bodies of water are visible from our apartment, we would simply stay home and enjoy the view. Unfortunately, there are also two big buildings obstructing our view right at the specific spots where the fireworks were. So we watched the pyrotechnics on TV and, from time to time, exclaimed, "I can see the top of that one!" as we looked out the window.

Today, before Brian's regular clinic appointment, we met Steve and Sharon Cohen and two of their kids for ice cream. We had a great time chatting away (and eating away, of course). Interestingly enough, I found myself surprised to learn that Steve is an attorney. I don't know what any of the other patients do for a living. We have met them, their health, their families, and their wonderful, shining personalities, without any of the trappings and pretension that often come with conversations that begin, "What do you do?"

Technically speaking, we're not supposed to socialize with other BMT patients, just as we weren't supposed to visit room to room in the hospital. But these are really some of the best friends we have out here, so we fudge it a little. Which, nine times out of ten, is fine. We won't think about the other one time.

After clinic, I popped up to see Don Prichard and walked a couple of laps with him and Cyndi. Things are still very up in the air, and they are just praying that this latest cocktail of treatments does the trick. This was the first time I had seen Don out of bed since before transplant, however, which was encouraging to me, at least.

So, that's what's new here. I am finding myself increasingly bored and lonely and often somewhat depressed. I thank God for how well Brian is doing, but that doesn't change how far away from our lives we are right now. So many of our friends and associates are on vacation, so the calls and whatnot from Pittsburgh have slowed. It's hard to accept that, although our lives are on hold, everyone else's continue.

Well, enough rambling. We are pulling for our friends and friends of

134

friends who are struggling through. Steve commented today that he thought the big key to Brian's success was that he "came to get a job done." He also said that Jack Sarfaty was in a class by himself. "Jack is Super-Jack" were his exact words. May all of you kick some butt getting your job done, too!

naomi

Date: Sun, 11 Jul 1999
Subject: Day +50: Half way there

I guess I should start by tying up a loose end or two from my last update. Apparently, I left the impression with some of you that I had dyed my hair purple. Relax. I may have lost it, but not that completely. "Bright burgundy" is a very natural looking color, particularly when put on hair as dark as mine. You would hardly notice the difference.

Now that Brian is off his nighttime hydration, he has been helping with little Ms. Sleepless at night. Brian's ability to get up with her has helped me retain what is left of my sanity.

This week we did a number of things that might be misconstrued as normal. On Wednesday, Joe gave us some "shore leave" and Brian and I went to the mall by ourselves. On Thursday, we went down to the market to buy fish and produce and Brian cooked up a yummy meal of salmon, pine nut couscous, and Chinese broccoli for our Internet friend, Cliff, who was over for dinner.

Friday, we brought in pizza and rented the movie *The Truman Show*. Brian gives it a thumbs up, while it left me so utterly disturbed that I couldn't find my thumbs when it was over. Yesterday, we went shopping for shirts for Brian. He has to wear long sleeves because he is very sensitive to the sun post-transplant, and he needed some more lightweight stuff given the weather. We also went to our favorite ice cream place with Mark but I refused to go into the park because I'm now afraid of the squirrels.

Today, we went to REI to buy a backpack carrier for Eve. I have it in my head that we're going to do some hiking while we're out here. We'll see, but the pack is probably a good thing to have anyway. In the afternoon, we walked about three miles to return our video and buy some fresh stuff for dinner with Brian carrying Eve in the pack on his back.

Our friend Bill, when he heard about this, asked if Brian was cross training. I said yes, that the BMT was kind of like wearing an extra bathing suit when you practice before a swim meet. It makes the exertion of the meet seem easy by comparison. Bill suggested Brian was involved in a triathlon — ten-mile hike, BMT, and parenting a baby who doesn't sleep through the night. In that order, of course, because it's the ascending order of difficulty.

Today I also visited Cyndi. Don, her husband, had a major mismatch with his donor (go get tested so no one else has to go through this!) and major complications both from that and from his conditioning regimen. He very nearly didn't make it, and still might not. However, I am pleased to report that he is off oxygen, his lungs appear to be improving slowly, and they are actually making noises about releasing him from the hospital. Cyndi has been with him 24 hours a day, 7 days a week for 35 days. I think she has left the hospital twice. Frankly, I think she needs out more than Don does.

I am finding that, perhaps because I have no one to be mad at about

136

being here or about Brian's health in general, customer service people at companies that have screwed up are getting a rather disproportionate chunk of my wrath. The billing department at the doctor's office, for example, managed to bill my insurance and then send me a threatening collection notice instead of a bill when my insurance denied coverage for Eve's appointment. Blam! Then they sent me a computer printout and some unintelligible forms when I asked for the bill. Double Blam! Our credit card keeps being denied and the company insists they can't fix it because they aren't denying it. Blam, blam, blam! I actually feel sorry for these poor, unsuspecting customer service people who are taking it on the chin from Caregiver Woman. But not very.

So, we are now at day 50 —half way up the stairs, so to speak. We will be back in touch whenever anything interesting happens, which might be Thursday after Brian's clinic appointment. In the meantime, we welcome your e-mails and calls and cards, which help break up the loneliness of being away from home. I thank you for being an audience for these e-mails, which help me put life in perspective and feel more connected to normalcy and to all of you, my wonderful support system.

naomi

Date: Thu, 16 Jul 1999
Subject: Day +54: Brian and the terrible, horrible, no good, very bad day

This morning, Brian woke up feeling like absolute cow pies. The increasing fatigue he had over the last few days grew to the point where taking a shower and getting dressed took two hours. He said he felt like his head was full of cotton. He was nauseous. He was lightheaded. In short, he felt punky. Or skunky. Or one of those other "unky" words.

Brian went up to clinic for his itra infusion, and I was to meet him for a social work appointment at 10. When I arrived, he was lying in a bed in the infusion room with the triage nurse standing over him. They had just done postural blood pressure and pulse — a check to see if his pressure drops and his pulse increases when he goes from lying to sitting to standing. His pressure was OK, but his pulse was 48 lying down (yes, you read that correctly) and 88 standing up. Bad. The nurse called Brian's doc and they ordered half a liter of IV fluids for him, since dehydration is one of the big causes of this phenomenon, otherwise known as postural hypotension.

As the fluids went into him, he went from being barely able to talk to me to somewhat animated, but he started to feel more nauseous, so they gave him some Benadryl®. His primary doctor came to see him and poked and prodded and said "hmm" a lot. After he left, Brian decided he needed to pee (500 ml of fluids will do that to you) and tried to get up. He nearly passed out, and when he came back from the bathroom he had a major shaking chill. He was under four thermal blankets fresh out of the warmer and still shaking.

The weird thing is, he had no fever. BMT patients who take steroids are sometimes unable to "express" a fever because their immune systems are too suppressed. But Brian isn't on systemic steroids.

At this point, the attending, Dr. S., who was Brian's inpatient attending in May, came around and asked him a lot of questions and said "hmm" a lot more. They decided he should hang out in the infusion room for a couple more hours to see if the chills came back or if he spiked a fever. They also drew blood cultures to see if there is some lurking infection that they can't detect through other means.

After two more hours and a Benadryl® induced nap, Brian felt much better, and the postural problem had gone away, so they sent him home. The minute he got home, he felt like dog doo (excuse me, cow pies, gotta keep my excrement straight here) once again. Just as I was getting really worried about this, we called for his counts today and found that his ANC had dropped by 50% since Monday. Yuck.

Late in the day Brian spoke with the team nurse, who has arranged for him to see Dr. S. again tomorrow. She said it's not uncommon for ANC to drop in the day 50-60 range, and also that the drop is consistent with a virus, which may be what's causing all of this in the first place. Although Brian went off his

138

beclomethasone on Tuesday, they feel it's a little early for his GVHD to be flaring up, so that's probably not it.

This was a really hard day emotionally for both Brian and me. Brian was absolutely terrified from the beginning that something really bad is wrong. He also feels, and I feel it too, that since he's been doing so well thus far that no one will believe him or care when he's sick. That's totally irrational, of course, but it's hard not to feel like people will say, "Ha, ha, told you so. That's what you get for being so healthy, you bonehead."

We both also found it very frustrating to have the doctors stand around and say "hmm." We find it a lot more useful when they say, "OK, here's a list of 75 things that could be going on, what they imply, and how we can differentiate them." The trouble is, a) most people really don't like that sort of thing and b) rumor has it that these doctors do have occasional other things to do besides spend 17 hours a day giving the Zikmund-Fishers a crash medical school course in BMT. Still, we are out of practice at noodging the docs to give us more information, and we need to get more into the swing of that if he's going to have actual medical issues again.

The odd thing is, although Brian clearly took a turn for the worse today, I don't feel the raging fear you might expect. Brian does, but I don't. I think that, when the going gets truly rough, I swing into action mode rather than allow myself the feelings that might otherwise go along with the situation. Today, I was too busy doing and asking to have time for thinking. Now, of course, as I read my own description of the day, it occurs to me that things aren't great. But I'm still in that action-denial mode, which is OK with me.

Tonight was the first night since Brian has been out of the hospital that he let me cook dinner, which will tell you how bad he is feeling. Not that my cooking would make him feel better, mind you. However, he did eat dinner and seems, to my practiced spousely eye, to be feeling quite a bit better. He's trying really hard to drink even more since dehydration seems to be at least part of the picture, but that's hard since he was already drinking more than three liters a day.

His nausea seems to be kicking up a tad, and he was very apprehensive about getting back on Ativan® to treat it. He doesn't want to get hooked again. I think I have convinced him that if he needs it he should take it and that, now that he knows how to safely come off, he won't have such a problem. We'll see.

"So, aside from that, Mrs. Lincoln, how was the play?" you ask.

The rest of the week has been great. My sister, Abby, came to visit for a couple of days, and we spent some time swimming and sight seeing and hanging out. It was great to see her, since we live several hundred miles away from each other even when I'm at home.

The latest on the "Brian hair watch" is that he has peach fuzz all over his face, including in places where he didn't used to have hair. His moustache makes him look like a junior high kid — not quite up to shaving but definitely something there. He has stubble on his head that is still quite loose. Tonight I pulled on one of the teeny tiny hairs on his shining bald head. When it came out, Brian said, "Hey, I was going to use that as a comb over for my bald spot!"

We have high hopes that tomorrow will be a better day. It's hard to retain the perspective that says, "You know, if he hadn't just had a BMT, we'd just say he had a low-grade bug."

I'm pleased to say I saw Don and Cyndi in outpatient today. Don was finally released from the hospital. Best to all and to all good days ahead. Some days are like this one. Even in Australia.

naomi

Brian awoke this morning feeling somewhat better than he did yester-day morning — perhaps only pigeon droppings instead of cow pies. The fatigue and aches and chills were gone, but the nausea and diarrhea had kicked up quite a bit. So he had worse symptoms, but didn't feel as sick, if that makes any sense.

He took half a mg of Ativan® and we headed up to clinic for his itra infu-sion and to see his doctors. He hadn't managed to down his pills before he left, which turned out to be a big mistake.

The nurse in the infusion room did posturals on him just like yesterday and he seemed in better shape. He was feeling really nauseous, however, and he decided that since oral Ativan® actually makes him feel worse briefly before it makes him feel better, he would try to take his cyclosporine before taking another half mg of Ativan®. Big mistake number two.

At this point, I, not being privy to the useful foreshadowing that you all get, toddled off to the waiting room and started schmoozing with Jack Sarfaty and his father and sister. When I returned, Brian was yacking away into an emesis basin. Great.

The nurse gave Brian some IV Ativan® and there was much discussion of whether he needed to repeat his cyclosporine dose. It was decided he didn't because no capsules had made their appearance in the aforementioned yak.

Brian's Fellow came to see him at this point. Now, you may recall that yesterday I was complaining that the doctors were not being terribly commu-nicative about what they thought was going on, and this was frustrating us. I specifically said I wanted a list of the possibilities and their implications. This complaint went out to my private mailing list and also to the Internet mailing list BMT-talk.

Well, I would bet serious bucks that Dr. V. either saw last night's mes-sage or was told about it. After talking to Brian about how he was feeling and about the drop in his ANC, he said, "Well, there are really four things that could be causing the drop in your counts." He then laid out the four things, which one he thought it was, and what the implications are of each. Much better.

They don't feel it's graft failure or infection. The best guess about what is going on at this point is that Brian is having a flare of his GVHD coupled with the random wanderings of counts post-transplant. It also happens that Bactrim®, which Brian takes two days a week to prevent pneumonia, can sup-press white counts. So they are taking him off the Bactrim® for the next two weeks.

After Dr. V. laid this all out for us, Dr. S., the attending, came by. She feels strongly that his GVHD is flaring and arranged for GI to see him in the afternoon. She gave him the option of starting prednisone today or holding on

141

until Monday when they can do another endoscopy which would qualify him for another round of beclomethasone, the study drug which he stopped taking for GVHD on Tuesday. Given the side effects of systemic steroids and the relative success he had with the bec before, she recommended and we agreed to wait until Monday and go for the bec.

Brian really seemed to be feeling much better this afternoon and wolfed down the traditional Shabbat dinner of a quarter-pounder from McDonald's this evening. He kept down his evening cyclosporine and played with Eve before bed. It is always possible that this isn't a flare at all and that it will go away on its own. Time will tell. We're not holding our breaths.

We're trying to keep perspective here. If this is the worst thing that happens during Brian's transplant, he got off extremely easily. However, if you've been reading my previous chronicles of this journey, you may have noticed that maintaining perspective is not always my strong suit. But I'm trying.

naomi

The good news is that Brian is feeling a good deal better than he was last week. He has nausea that comes in waves, but between the waves he really feels fine.

Clinic today brought some interesting conversations. As you may recall, Dr. S., his current attending, was his attending inpatient when he had to ask for special permission to get Hershey bars. Well, today we presented her with a Hershey bar, the last of the stash. OK, actually it was going to be the last of the stash, but in a fit of stress last Thursday I ate the last of the stash, so this was a fresh, newly purchased one. She thought this was a riot and gave Brian a big hug.

We talked about a lot of things at clinic today. Dr. S. is not convinced that he's having a GVHD flare, and, if he is, it's mild and kind of chronic. She floated the idea that, if the endoscopy didn't find GVHD, Brian might go off the itraconazole entirely and see if perhaps that's what's causing his nausea. That wouldn't explain the chills and dizziness from last week, but neither would GVH, and those symptoms seem to have resolved themselves.

We also talked a lot about childcare options for the fall. Probably, were Brian not ill, we would put Eve in daycare when I go back to work. But daycare centers are full of germs which kids pass back and forth and then bring home to immunocompromised Daddies. Also, the aforementioned Daddy has long been toying with the idea of being a part-time at-home parent, but changing diapers is problematic for immunocompromised patients.

Dr. S. feels that it's OK for Brian to be Eve's caregiver if he feels up to it, including changing diapers. She also thinks that daycare should be avoided if possible as long as Brian is on cyclosporine, which current predictions have at four months to a year. So we think we are going to have Brian care for Eve two days a week and do some kind of nanny arrangement as yet to be determined the other three days.

I tried to engage Dr. S. in a discussion of "the plan" for the next several weeks, but she wouldn't bite. Too much is currently up in the air to go there. This is hard for me because, slowly, the people we met here are getting ready to go home. Most of them are way further along than Brian, but some are not, and that's frustrating. As much as I know it's not a race and that the important thing is for him to be healthy, I really want to go home. And watching others go makes me feel like we'll be left here all alone which, in a transplant center as big as this one, would be quite something!

In the waiting room today we were talking to Jack Sarfaty and I said something about "hating" somebody who is getting ready to go home. This woman is probably a month ahead of Brian, and she's doing really well. Jack didn't even look up. He just said, "Your turn's coming." I don't know why, but that really helped.

As Dr. V., the Fellow, was leaving the room at the end of Brian's clinic appointment today, the nurse came in with Brian's counts. Because he was having the endoscopy today, they did a blood draw to be sure his platelets were high enough. All of his counts were down, which merited Dr. V. coming back to talk to us about them. As he said, "Why should I tell you I am not worried? You are worried." I think they're getting to know me around here.

Basically, no one knows what is causing this and everyone agrees that the trend is disturbing, but no one is worried because the levels aren't that low as yet. The most likely thing is that his counts are just bouncing around and they will bounce back up. Another possibility is that the Bactrim® is suppressing his counts, which is why they've taken him off it. The most worrisome possibility is, of course, that his graft is failing. However, this is really unlikely. There is no point, at this stage, in doing another marrow to look at his graft because, given the levels he's at, it would probably be inconclusive. So we just have to wait for another couple of weeks until his day 75 marrow, by which time we hope that his counts will at least have stabilized. You know how much I love waiting.

I would be lying if I told you I wasn't terrified about this. I can tell you all the reasons why this might be fine and normal, but it just doesn't feel fine and normal. I want things to be going up, up, up! I did talk to two other families today who had similar drops around this time, however, so that kind of helped.

Uncertainty is very draining. Illness and hard times we can handle, as long as we know everything will be OK in the end. It seems so surreal to, at one and the same time, feel like he is so healthy we should be able to go home and fear that his graft is failing and he might not make it at all. For the first time since he was in the hospital, I'm again contemplating the possibility that he might die. I liked not contemplating it better.

Brian had his endoscopy this afternoon. They had somewhat more trouble sedating him this time. In the middle of trying to put him under, his pulse ox, the measure of oxygen in his blood, tanked, so they put him on oxygen and had to keep telling him to breathe, which was a little scary for me. He, of course, doesn't remember this. He wasn't quite as asleep as he was last time, therefore, and when they were done he talked about how hard it was to get the scope in. But now he doesn't remember that, either.

His endoscopy looked pretty normal. They saw some red streaking, but the doc said it wasn't consistent in appearance or location with GVH. They took some biopsies, since sometimes things look normal when they aren't, but even I could tell the difference between the last one and this one in how healthy his stomach looked. We should have biopsy results tomorrow afternoon or perhaps on Wednesday.

We saw Cliff and Carol Slaughterbeck briefly today. Carol was at clinic

144

for another dose of the experimental anti-cancer vaccine. They were kind enough to bring us all sorts of leftover Hickman supplies from when Carol had her Hickman, which will save us some money. Carol looks fantastic and stood out rather starkly at the outpatient clinic as the only person there with hair!

Carol found a lump on her collarbone last week and the docs seem to think it might be a cuff that stayed in her chest when they removed her Hickman. The other obvious possibility, and one that scares us all, is that it's a relapse of her breast cancer. Her doctors are so unconcerned they aren't even going to biopsy. I hope they're right!

Meanwhile, back at the ranch, we had kind of a lazy weekend. Mark and I went to the track on Saturday and each played our "system." His is to bet on horses with trainers and jockeys with good records. Mine is to bet on horses with clever names. Brian also asked us to place some bets for him. His system is to bet favorites late in the day, which has actually been scientifically proven to work for reasons I won't go into here. Of course, Brian was the only one whose system actually worked because he's a geek. I lost plenty of money and had a great time. Being away from Eve for that length of time made me feel like an absolute wild woman.

Ms. Eve was kind enough to have two consecutive nights of no nursing, causing me to have two consecutive nights of not having to get out of bed. If you don't have small kids, that may not seem like much, but after 13 and a half months of getting up anywhere from one to seven times a night, none seems like a major holiday! Of course, I keep going to bed way too late so I'm still totally pooped.

Thanks all for your care and concern. Hearing from all of you is what keeps us going. Watch this space.

naomi

Well, once again, no news is no news. Brian's biopsy results did not come back this afternoon, so we're expecting them in the morning. I don't know why I keep expecting lab results to come back when they say they will, because I don't think that has ever happened in this entire transplant process. You'd think I'd learn.

Meanwhile, Brian felt pretty weird today. "OK," you're saying, "he's a pretty weird guy. What do you mean?" This morning, he found that his feet were tingling as though they were falling asleep. He went up to clinic for his infusion thinking he was going to report this new side effect, but it went away. However, when he came home he felt quite lightheaded and seemed kind of out of it. The problem with this is that Brian tends to be very quiet and withdrawn when he doesn't feel well, so it's hard to tell if he's actually disoriented or just being himself. Later in the day, his diarrhea started up again. He was also complaining of muscle fatigue.

Brian reported all of this to his team nurse and then, frankly, lost it. Which is OK, in my opinion, because if I were in his shoes I'd lose it a heck of a lot more often. Brian feels, as do I in some ways, that everything is headed in the wrong direction. Instead of starting out sick and getting healthier, he started out healthy and seems to be getting sicker. This has an ominous feel to it, even if it doesn't signify much. Brian also feels that it's hard for him to communicate the real changes in his physical condition because, objectively, he still is in great shape for someone at this stage post-transplant. But he knows he's not doing as well as he was and he feels like no one believes him.

Part of the problem is that Brian doesn't want to seem like a whiner, so when people ask him how he's doing, he always starts with something positive. For a teacher conducting a parent conference, this is great. "Johnny has perfect attendance" comes before "He keeps stabbing the other kindergartners with scissors." But for a patient communicating physical deterioration, this isn't the greatest idea. This afternoon, he talked on the phone to Moreen about how frustrated he felt trying to communicate how bad he feels, but when she asked him how he was feeling, he said, "Pretty good!"

We hope to have more answers, or at least some different questions, sometime tomorrow. I will keep you posted.

Meanwhile, on the home front, a friend in Pittsburgh who has a daughter a few months older than Eve has agreed, on a trial basis, to watch Eve three days a week when I return to work September 1. This is a tremendous load off of our minds because it means we don't have to do nanny hunting at a distance.

Thanks once again to all for your e-mails. I was telling Brian tonight how horrendously unloved I felt and then started going through the list of all the

146

people who have written in the last 24 hours. It's long, and much appreciated, even if it only puts a dent in the loneliness and isolation. I suspect that the loneliness and isolation actually have very little to do with how alone or isolated I really am. At some point, my psyche just had to give out.

naomi

Brian woke up this morning with some pretty nasty diarrhea. Around here, diarrhea pretty much equals "need to see doctor before you can go home from clinic," so we waited around most of the morning for this to occur.

Brian's biopsy from his endoscopy came back "equivocal." On the one hand, it wasn't quite normal. On the other hand, there was only the slightest hint of GVHD visible. It's impossible to say whether this is a relapse of GVHD or whether it never went away in the first place, because they didn't do an endoscopy while he was still on the beclomethasone. However, given that he responded well to bec in the past and that he is having all these yucky GI symptoms, they are putting him back on the bec for another 28-day course. They can't guarantee that it will work or that the GVHD won't come back when he goes off it in four weeks, but we're going to give it another try.

Dr. V. spent a long time talking to us today and trying to reassure us that all of this is normal ups and downs of transplant. It's so hard, since Brian was really only having ups until last week. I said to Dr. V. that "he felt so much better 10 days ago" and he said, "I think he's going to feel so much better in 10 days." We tried to get that in writing, but no go.

Brian has a new attending starting today. Usually they rotate once a month, but apparently someone was covering for someone else for two weeks, so we get Dr. H. for the next two weeks and then they rotate again. That will make 4 attendings in 7 weeks, which I think is a little disruptive but nobody asked me! We didn't get to meet Dr. H. today, which doesn't add to that wonderful feeling of continuity.

This afternoon we had ice cream with Steve and Sharon Cohen. Actually, all of us had ice cream except Steve, who has prednisone-induced diabetes. My sense is that giving up certain foods is by far the hardest part of transplant for him so far. Steve and Sharon, however, have absolutely the greatest attitude about this whole process. It always helps to see them, because they keep their eye on what is important — getting better — whereas I keep my eye on things like whether Brian will win the contest for "BMT Patient of the Year" or something.

After Eve's nap, we went for a walk around the Japanese Gardens at the arboretum. This was a better idea in principle than in practice, since we couldn't let Eve run around because she wanted to hurl herself into the pond to catch the carp. However, Brian and I got into a lengthy discussion of my future, which was very thought provoking.

I've been thinking more and more that perhaps the classroom isn't really where I'm meant to be. I like my job as a special education teacher, and I don't think I'm bad at it, but I'm not passionate about it anymore. Now, I also

148

haven't done it in 16 months, so I may be surprised how I feel when I get back in September, we'll see. But I also feel like this experience with Brian, from the donor search to the insurance debacle to the transplant itself and all that I've learned, has changed me in some fundamental way that needs to be put to good use. I can't imagine absorbing this experience and all that I now know and pocketing it and going back and not doing anything with it. I'm just not sure how I can do something with it, or if it actually requires a career change or just some refocusing of my volunteer time or what.

In the short term, I owe the Board of Education at least one more year in return for the extended leave they gave me to care for Eve and Brian, so no decisions are imminent.

Well, as my friend Michelle would say, "Enough about me. Let's talk about you. What do you think of me?"

Thanks for all your warm thoughts and encouragement — we need it. We're hanging in and you do the same!

naomi

Chapter 7:
That's the News and We Are Out of Here!

Date: Thu, 22 Jul 1999
Subject: Day +61: Movin' on up

Yesterday I was chatting with Chuck, the receptionist at the clinic, and he said I looked blue and he wanted to help. I said, "Make Brian better." He turned to his computer and pantomimed typing "better" and then turned to me and asked, "What would you like his counts to be?" We had a nice laugh.

This afternoon I called Chuck to get Brian's counts. All of Brian's counts were way, way up. I told Chuck I loved him and thanked him for making it better. Later in the afternoon, I brought Chuck some chocolate covered grahams from Starbucks in celebration and, frankly, in thanks for how nice and competent and wonderful he is to everyone here. He gave me a high five. It is a better day.

Brian is still having waves of nausea, and is trying to be more proactive with the Ativan®. He started up the bec again last night, so it's too early to really be making a difference. We will probably never know what sent his counts into the sewer, but it's nice to see them headed in the right direction.

This morning I had a nice long chat on the phone with Mary, a woman I know from the Internet whose daughter, Katy, was transplanted in Texas a few weeks before Brian. We both were feeling pretty low I think. There comes a point where you feel so blah all the time that it stops having any content. The situation just stinks so egregiously that you have to feel yucky, even if there isn't one particular reason.

It was good to talk to Mary because she's very down to earth and doesn't try to give you stupid self-assured advice or play "can you top this" with caregiver misery. Misery is misery. Brian's counts did put me in a somewhat better frame of mind, though. Also, frankly, I think I needed to wallow a little to get it out of my system.

This evening we went out with our volunteer family. Eve had a great time on this excursion. She particularly enjoyed the part where I would try to get her to make the sound of a hippopotamus chewing gum ("grum grum grum grum grum grum grum," for those of you who don't read Dr. Seuss), one of her favorite and best tricks, and she would look at me blankly. Finally, late in the evening on about the 86th time I had asked her what the sound of a hippopotamus chewing gum is, she looked at me, shook her head, and said, "no, no, no." I can see her in therapy in 20 years saying, "My mom never really loved me for who I am. All she wanted was to show her friends how I could say 'grum grum grum.'"

Best to all, and thanks for your support.

naomi

Date: Mon, 26 Jul 1999
Subject: Day +65: Homeward bound (?)

On Friday, the side of Brian's Hickman catheter which they draw blood out of conked out entirely. The catheter splits into two tubes at the end. One has a red cap and one a white cap to distinguish them. Certain medications go into one side and certain into the other side and blood draw pretty much always comes out of the red side.

IV itraconazole, the antifungal that Brian has been on, goes into the red side and is really viscous and tends to gum up the line. Brian has been madly flushing that side for weeks but finally it died. Stuff goes in, but nothing comes out.

Brian's doctors felt this was a good time to see if he could stop the IV itra and start taking the liquid again. In short, the answer is no. He tried it on Friday and barfed it back up immediately. They took him off the IV and told him to try oral once over the weekend. Well, he tried on Sunday and, as he put it, barely made the bowl. Oral itra is not going to happen. So, as of his clinic appointment today, Brian officially withdrew from the clinical trial of itra and will begin fluconazole, the standard antifungal, tomorrow. It comes in pill form and he only has to take it for ten more days.

Aside from the itra barfage, Brian is feeling pretty good. He is mostly Ativan®-free and only feels nauseous if his stomach is completely empty. He is going through crackers, pretzels, and Chex Mix at an alarming rate. More than one person has suggested he has morning sickness. Now that would be an interesting side effect of BMT!

His counts today were pretty much identical to Thursday's. Stable is good, we don't need up so much as absence of down.

The biggest news from clinic today is that they are talking about sending Brian home. I mean home, as in Pittsburgh home. As in home home. As in yay.

The deal appears to be this: presuming no new complications (and that is always a possibility), Brian will begin his day 80 work-up next week. If all goes well, we will go home somewhere around day 82. Now, as I said, all things are approximate. And if he gets sicker or anything unexpected happens, all bets are off. But we are very excited at the prospect of heading out of here.

Brian and I stopped by the hospital today to see Suzanne and Dick McKee. Suzanne is another one of my BMT-talk buddies, and Dick just checked into the hospital today for his transplant. Dick was actually up and walking with a Foley catheter in. Brian's comment was that, with an attitude like that, he was going to do great. Way to go Dick and Suzanne, keep up the good work!

Meanwhile, back at the ranch, my brother Abe and my niece Wendy

153

were here for the weekend. One of the neat things about this trip has been getting to see my siblings without their entire families in tow. Don't get me wrong, I love all my nieces and nephews, but it's very different to interact with my siblings when they have a little time to be people and not just parents.

Brian and I are slowly wading through the ever-increasing number of decisions we need to make about life at home, from what volunteer and job-related commitments we are going to keep to whether we are going to buy a second car. We avoided these decisions before we came out here because we couldn't look past the transplant. We didn't want to look at what would happen if things went badly, and we couldn't bring ourselves to have enough hope to plan for things going well. But now, plans are slowly falling into place. It's hard to believe that in only a little more than a month I'll be back to working full time.

Going home seems very surreal. How can we possibly transition from being here, where pretty much all our attention is on Brian and getting him well, to being home, where we actually have a life? What if we can't manage to have that life? What does it feel like to just get up every day and go about your business without worrying about test results and whether your sweetie is going to barf today? I don't remember.

Best to all, and hope to see many of you soon!

naomi

Date: Fri, 30 Jul 1999
Subject: Day +69

There isn't a whole lot medical to report. Brian hasn't seen a doctor since Monday and is feeling pretty good. He is having some trouble sleeping, which makes him grouchy, which makes me grouchy, which makes Eve grouchy. We're quite a bunch. Brian's counts are stable and his spirits, other than the above sleepless grouchiness, are pretty good.

We went outlet shopping on Wednesday with his mom and Aunt Shirley. Brian found the day very hard. Temperature changes (outside to inside air conditioning) are particularly uncomfortable for him, and he got pretty tired. However, to put this in perspective, he was up bright and early yesterday morning helping Mark move.

I hate watching Brian dissolve as the day goes on. I want him to feel 100% all the time. He is supposed to be the marrow stud, doing better than anyone's wildest dreams at all times. It's hard to cut him a little slack and say that he's entitled to be a tad pooped once in a while.

Eve and I stopped by the hospital yesterday to see Dick and Suzanne. Dick had a rough time with his chemo but looked downright terrific yesterday. I like spending time with Suzanne because, in addition to being a nice person, she's every bit as crazy and paranoid as I am. So we both know we can say what's on our mind, even if it sounds nuts, and the other one will understand.

Suzanne worries incessantly about bringing germs into Dick's room, from what footwear to wear in the family shower to who is allowed to visit. This was never a huge issue for me. However, I worry incessantly that Brian's health is going to be "jinxed" by too much good news and that every word I write in these updates will offend someone or make them stop caring about me. So Suzanne and I are kind of even in the nuttiness department. It's nice to have a soul mate.

The big news here is that Valerie Vernon, the Pink Power Ranger on FOX's "Power Rangers: Lost Galaxy," who is herself a BMT patient, is donating some autographed pictures and a toy to be auctioned on the Internet to benefit the Brian Zikmund-Fisher Fund at the HLA Registry. Brian and I have been busily scurrying around creating a press release about this. Yes, I know this isn't the blockbuster news story of the week, but it never hurts to try! Brian also put together a hotsy-totsy new webpage about the fund. Looks like we may have found a joint project after all!

Tonight, we went to Steve and Sharon Cohen's house for Shabbat dinner. Yes, I know that that's a major violation of the rules, but people will just have to get over it. It was funny, because Steve kept assuring Brian that all the food was properly prepared and that he could eat everything, which we thought was pretty obvious.

Steve and Brian had a good time comparing methods for getting a yarmulke to stay on a bald head (apparently, suede yarmulkes and a little sweat works nicely). Eve had a wonderful time, and spent most of the evening, when she wasn't eating, trying to kiss Steve's seven-year-old son, much to his dismay. It was nice to have such a normal, social evening for a change.

Well, that's the news here. I hope everyone has a wonderful weekend!

naomi

Date: Sun, 1 Aug 1999
Subject: Day +71: Bid, bid, BID!

The auctions for The Brian Zikmund-Fisher Fund at the HLA Registry Foundation have begun! For those of you not on my Internet mailing list, I have been much enjoying your bewildered questions about how the heck I know the Pink Power Ranger! Her fiancé subscribes to the same BMT list as I do. Not surprisingly, the media hasn't exactly pounced on this as yet, but it was worth a try.

Brian is having a rough weekend. His diarrhea is back and that doesn't feel too good. After several rounds of this, however, he knew it was coming and was able to push fluids preemptively so he didn't get his usual dizziness, etc. It's weird how these symptoms, which a year ago would have been stomach flu and a month ago would have caused panic, have now become a regular part of our lives. Not only can Brian feel it coming, but he knows what to do to keep it from being too bad. I guess it's good to be in tune with your body, but I wish he didn't feel like he needed to be.

I saw Suzanne yesterday and we spent more time being paranoid together. Dick's doing great. Suzanne doesn't want people traipsing into Dick's room, so Suzanne and Eve and I hung out in the family lounge. She has a lot on her mind, obviously, so I'm pretty amazed at how much time she has for me and my stupid obsessions.
You'd think I'd be getting less stressed as the time to leave approaches, but that's not true. First of all, I'm afraid we aren't really going to leave. And second of all, going home means shifting a lot of the burden for worrying about Brian from the doctors and nurses to me. However, being a consummate worrier, I think I'm probably equal to the task.

Thank you, everyone!

naomi

Date: Mon, 2 Aug 1999
Subject: Day +72

Today was the first day of Brian's "departure work-up." Basically, they have to look back at every square inch of his body, in and out, and figure out if it looks substantially worse than when they checked it before the transplant. Today, he had three tests: a Schirmer's eye test, a bone marrow aspiration and a skin biopsy.

The eye test is a test for chronic GVHD in his eyes. Some people don't produce enough tears after transplant. Our friend Jack Sarfaty has been dealing with this and getting all sorts of treatments for his eyes and skin. Anyway, for this test, they put some soothing drops in Brian's eyes and then put little pieces of paper in his eyes under the lid. If his eyes water and soak the paper, he passes. He passed.

The bone marrow aspiration is to see whether there is any sign of the MDS, what percentage of a normal, healthy person's cell count he has and what percentage of the cells are donor cells versus his old marrow. These results will take 10-14 days.

The skin biopsy looks for signs of GVHD of the skin. He had one as an inpatient, which was negative, but they want to know if anything has sprung up in the meantime. Those results should be back in a couple of days.

Brian also had a fasting cholesterol and triglycerides test. Cyclosporine can massively elevate both of these things, so they want to make sure he's not ripe for a heart attack. They weren't expecting the levels to be normal, just not too high. Well, lo and behold, they were normal. It helps that Brian's triglycerides were absurdly low before transplant. The nurse said she had never seen normal cholesterol and triglycerides post-transplant, ever.

Brian also had his weekly clinic appointment today. They are promising us that, should nothing unforeseen happen, we can leave the week of the 16th. They feel that the diarrhea at the current level is not worrisome, so long as he continues to be able to eat and drink around it. Frankly, they're hoping it will just go away by itself.

I am starting to get all panicky about leaving Eve when I go back to work, not because I distrust her caregivers in any way but because she's been my security blanket for the last 14 months and it's hard to say goodbye, even for a little while each day. I know, I know, thousands of people before me have done this and their kids didn't grow up to be ax murderers. There's always a first time.

The great Power Rangers auction is shaping up nicely, and I'm getting a real kick out of watching it go. I e-mailed some other celebrities whose lives have been touched by cancer over the weekend, and got one tentative yes to donate an autograph. I don't want to spill the beans before the commitment's final, but, well, you know the 3 Tenors? He's the one whose name you can

158

never remember. If anyone has any other ideas of people I should contact, please let me know!

It feels really good to be doing something positive and potentially successful around bone marrow transplant. After feeling for so long that this situation was so complex and rare that no one understood what we were going through, it's nice to do something from the opposite side of that coin. Because no one understands this stuff, no one does much about it. We're in the rare position of being able to do something constructive because we know about it. As the saying goes, when life gives you lemons, make lemonade.

The clock is hopefully ticking on this phase of this journey. We're starting to ship sweaters and books home, so this may all come to an end someday.

naomi

Date: Tue, 3 Aug 1999
Subject: Day +73

Today, Brian had his departure exam at Oral Medicine. They asked him tons of questions about his mouth — pain, sensitivity to heat, cold, or spices, thickened saliva, you name it. The only thing he has is the very slightest bit of thickened saliva in the morning, which he probably had before but never thought about it. Everything looked pretty good.

The only new thing that came out of this visit was a "what to look for at home" instruction for Brian. He is to report promptly any new sores, dryness, or sensitivity to spices, which might indicate GVHD in his mouth. He is also supposed to look at all parts of his mouth every two weeks or so in the mirror to make sure there aren't any weird looking patches or lines. He is not supposed to have any routine dental work including cleaning for 6 to 12 months, but he is supposed to have an oral exam and, if needed, x-rays in four or five months just to make sure there isn't anything icky brewing in there. Icky is a highly technical medical term.

Life here continues to be life. I know it sounds like absolutely nothing is happening around here and like we're pretty bored. This is completely accurate. I never thought we'd get to the point when we could say we were coasting, but it does seem that way. Still, we're coasting thousands of miles from home. And although we're making lots of plans to come home, we're not there yet.

Eve's word of the day is uh-oh, which she says whenever she drops something. Unfortunately, she decided to try to create as many opportunities to practice saying this as possible. It was a long but very cute day.

naomi

160

Date: Fri, 6 Aug 1999
Subject: Day +76

Yesterday, Brian continued his "departure work-up" with a visit to nutrition and a pulmonary function test.

At nutrition, we found that his weight is down again, probably due to the diarrhea he's been having. The nutritionist told us she doesn't think, as the docs do, that it's spicy food that's upsetting his gut but rather soluble fiber. She suggested that he lay off the mountains of vegetables contained in the stir-fry and curry which seem to wreak havoc with his bowels and try more insoluble fiber like white rice, bananas, and applesauce.

She also assured us that the ribbing Brian has been taking about his diet, which has made us feel like the doctors and nurses all think he's insane for trying to eat this stuff, is actually veiled jealousy that we actually have time to cook it. We're thinking we should cook lunch for the team sometime before we leave.

Since that appointment, Brian has been trying to be a tad more practical about his diet and to watch his fiber intake. It's funny that all the things that are good for you any other time are no-nos after a transplant. Anyway, it seems to be working because he reports no stomach trouble at all today.

After nutrition, we reported to pulmonary. They redid all of the tests they did when he first arrived here to see how much decrease in lung function he's had due to the transplant. The short answer was, not much.

I wasn't present at his first pulmonary function test, so it was fun for me to watch. Essentially, they have him breathe into a big machine in various patterns — normally, then as deep as he can and blow out as far as he can, then in as fast as he can and out as fast as he can, then hyperventilate, then breathe pure oxygen, etc. There are breaks after each of these tests, and each one creates a neat graph on a computer screen. Of course, I have no clue what the graph signifies, but it's cool.

Anyway, all but one of the tests showed his lungs were in as good shape as before, and most of them showed he was actually doing slightly better! This was rather unexpected. We expected him to lose some lung function during transplant and slowly gain it back, but Brian has apparently used the BMT as a rare physical training opportunity.

Yesterday evening, I had a flash of realization that I had forgotten to call for Brian's counts. I think it's a telling thing that I wasn't so obsessed with them for once. I called this morning and, lo and behold, his counts were all down a fair amount, which is what I get for not obsessing. Since he had a marrow done on Monday there's nothing to do but wait for the results of that to find out if the count dipping is due to anything more serious than the meds he's taking. In the meantime, I'll return to obsessing. I'm good at it.

Today, Brian had no appointments and so took the afternoon to go see

161

"Star Wars Episode I." He went by himself because a) Eve doesn't go for that stuff and b) after 20+ years I am finally comfortable enough with myself to admit that I hate Star Wars. Anyway, he went to this enormous, 500 seat, 68 foot screen theater for a 1 o'clock matinee. He said there were only about 60 people there, which was the point of doing it this way — no crowds.

We've been spending our spare time watching the auctions for the BZ-F Fund go up (which, yes, is like watching the grass grow, but I'm just tickled that we did it at all). We have no plans for the weekend other than to watch the Blue Angels, the military stunt pilot team, practice and perform in a show that goes directly over our building.

naomi

Date: Mon, 9 Aug 1999
Subject: Day +79: t-9

Today's festivities at the clinic began with a brief visit to nutrition, where Brian's regular nutritionist was unavailable and the woman covering kept flipping back in the book and looking at Brian's calorie counts and saying, "Wow!"

Brian's diarrhea is completely gone and he's back to eating like a horse, so his weight has started to come back a little. He still weighs less than when I met him. For those of you who might not have calculated it, this means he can actually turn sideways and not be seen. In all seriousness, he looks thin but not scrawny, although he doesn't have a whole lot more body fat to work with.

We then proceeded to Brian's clinic appointment, where his Fellow came in and said, "We're concerned because you are planning to leave next week and you're coming off the beclomethasone next week, and what if your GVHD flares while you're flying? Maybe you should stay an extra week." This went over like an absolute lead balloon.

I immediately and without thinking about it switched into my "excuse me while I politely take a shovel to the back of your head" mode. I pointed out that, two weeks ago when they told us he could leave the week of the 16th and last week when they said, and I quote, "We made that promise and we're sticking to it," they certainly knew he was stopping the bec on the 18th. It wasn't like it snuck up on them. I suggested that if they were so concerned about a flare, that they send him home before he stopped the bec so, if he had a flare, he would not be traveling at the time. This also went over like a lead balloon.

I was pretty ticked off. You have to understand that I am returning to work full time after more than 17 months of maternity/family leave on September 1, and the notion of getting back into town only a week before or less does not please me. I also felt that this problem was foreseeable and they shouldn't have made a promise they couldn't keep. It would be one thing if something new came up — I understand you can't ever foresee everything — but they knew about this! Grrrrrr.

Anyway, at this point Dr. W., the attending, came in. He looked Brian over, sat down and said, "Look, the choice is to send you home on Wednesday the 18th or for you to stay another week. I don't think you're dying to stay another week. Do you want to go home on the 18th?" And that was that. Unless (and it is not uncommon, mind you) Brian spikes a fever or some other problem crops up, he will be released from the center's care on the 17th and go home the 18th.

But wait, you knew there had to be a catch.

We flew out here on Frequent Flyer tickets. When I called to change them from the 30th to the 18th, I was informed that there were no seats available on the 18th. The only seats they could give us were at 8 AM on the 17th

163

(which would be before he was discharged, which would be bad) or on the 22nd (which might well be in the middle of a GVHD flare, which would be really bad).

I explained to each of three successive departments that Brian is a cancer patient, that he needs treatment on the 17th here and on the 19th in Pittsburgh, that flying standby is not OK, and that I had a hard time believing they didn't have any seats on any flights going anywhere that could connect to Pittsburgh on the 18th, seeing as how Pittsburgh is a major hub for the airline.

Number one of these morons had the audacity to tell me that "this isn't really a medical issue. Why can't he just stay out there?" Let's just say it was a very good thing we were on the phone, because otherwise I would be in jail doing time for assault with a cordless phone. The number two moron actually had the nerve to tell me I couldn't speak to her supervisor because she already had spoken to her for me and they weren't going to help me.

When I arrived at moron number three, lo and behold there was indeed a seat available. But, of course, it was a "revenue" seat and not a frequent flyer seat, so to get it we would have to pay $900. I stamped my widdle foot some more and, after literally an hour and a half on the phone, I got them to agree to give Brian that seat for free if they could confirm my story with both the center here and his doctor in Pittsburgh. What jerks.

So Eve and I will be returning to Pittsburgh the morning of Tuesday the 17th, and Brian will follow the afternoon of the 18th. I do not cherish the thought of flying 7 hours (because of course this isn't a direct flight) by myself with a 14-month-old, but you do what you gotta do. Brian gets a direct flight. I hate him.

The other news of the day is that the initial results of Brian's bone marrow biopsy were normal — no sign of MDS. We don't have the percentages on how much is donor and how much is him yet. That will come this weekend. We have a lot to do between now and next Tuesday, and we're feeling a little overwhelmed.

You will also be pleased to know that the charity auction is over, so I can stop talking about it for a minute and a half. Brian and I spent over an hour yesterday putting color into the fonts on the fund website and having such conversations as, "Make it darker. No not that dark. No lighter. No more medium. No not that medium, eeewww." We're done, thank God, and maybe we can leave it alone for a while. But it would make me happy if everyone would check it out so I would feel like there was a purpose to doing this, even though there probably wasn't. It's at www.bzffund.org.

I promise I will stop obsessing now. You know how it goes, when you can't fix the important things, you obsess about the little ones.

Thanks to everyone and I hope to be e-mailing from Pittsburgh soon!

naomi
164

Date: Thu, 12 Aug 1999
Subject: Day +82: My candle burns at both ends

It is only 11 AM here and I already think my day warrants an update, which should give you an idea of what kind of day we're having.

Monday night, someone from my BMT-talk list suggested I contact an organization that flies cancer patients on extra seats on corporate jets, to see if they could get us all home on the same flight on Wednesday.

My day began today with being awakened at 6:45 AM by a call from this organization. Ever hear of a time change, people? In the first place, they didn't have a flight to put us on. But even if they did, they said, they wouldn't have because, for adult patients, they will only fly one adult escort. We couldn't take Eve.

Now, I know intellectually that, whether or not this policy makes sense, it makes no practical difference because, if they don't have a flight to put us on, their being unwilling to fly Eve is kind of beside the point. However, this conversation just put me over the edge. I have had it. I'm exhausted, I'm stressed and I'm frustrated. I know that all these special programs and promotions and discounts are there to help the patients, and that's great and how it should be. But being the caregiver isn't exactly a walk in the park either. I don't think we've abused any systems in this experience, and I just need a break on this one thing. Having spent the hour and a half yelling at the airline on Monday just to get them to cough up the seat for Brian, I don't really want to hear about how no one is going to help me because I have a baby. If I didn't have the baby, I wouldn't need the help.

I said to Brian that somehow it seems that at moments like these in other people's lives, a miracle occurs and someone swoops down from on high and solves their problem, so why doesn't that happen to me? He pointed out that no one would send out a breathless e-mail about the time they had a huge problem that didn't get solved. You only hear about the good stuff.

In the history of the free world, this is not the biggest thing. It's just the biggest thing to me. It's the end of four months of stress, and I just don't want to cope. This is supposed to be a happy, triumphant return, and I feel like they're stealing that from me. I can't deal. Maybe some of you other caregivers out there can relate.

After this occurred, Brian was trying to cheer me up and got into a tickle fight with Eve, who obligingly giggled, laughed, and kicked his chest, pulling out his Hickman slightly. So then we had to run up to the clinic and get it checked. It's OK, but again, not what we needed.

Actually, what I really need is a nap.

naomi

Date: Sun, 15 Aug 1999
Subject: Day +85

Let's start with the burning question that's on everyone's mind. Now, for most BMT patients at this point, it's "What were the results of your marrow test?," but for us it's "Did you figure out how you're getting home?"

Dealing with the airline has been like that old Vaudeville sketch where the guy says, "I'd like coffee and a sweet roll" and the waitress says, "We don't have any sweet rolls" and the guy says, "OK, then I'll have tea and a sweet roll," etc. Except in our case, they said, "We can get you home on the 17th" and we said "We need to go on the 18th" and they said, "OK, well, how about the 17th, then" and on it went. And on, and on, and on.

Yesterday, my cousin's wife was here and she took a crack at it. After a full hour on the phone, she got them to propose, and here's the shocker, that we go home on the 17th. Great. Their solution was that Brian move his appointments to facilitate this. Thanks a bunch for your care and compassion for the sick.

Today we had our summary conference with Dr. W. and told him the story, and he said that he felt it was important that we all go home together. I'm glad someone thought it was! Nice to know I'm not totally insane. Or at least not on this one issue. So he arranged for Brian's last appointment on Tuesday to be moved to tomorrow, Monday so we can leave here together first thing Tuesday morning and arrive in Pittsburgh around 6 PM.

Our meeting with Dr. W. lasted about 90 minutes and ran through every-thing about Brian's current clinical status and the recommendations for the months ahead. No one could ever accuse Dr. W. of skimming over anything!

Brian's marrow is 80% cellular, right what they expect at this point, and about 97% donor marrow (above 95% is A+). All of the cell lines are engrafting. There is no sign of MDS so HA HA to you stupid fate! Oops, sorry, I'm back now. His cytogenetics, the molecular look at any mutations in his marrow cells, are all normal. Everything looks great.

Brian's skin biopsy was positive for graft-versus host disease, which was something of a surprise since he has no symptoms in his skin. They are classifying him as having "subclinical chronic GVHD of the skin," and they aren't going to treat it. However, given the diarrhea and nausea he continues to have, it seems likely that his GVHD of the gut is still going. If so, it will probably rear its ugly head in the next couple of weeks after he finishes his beclomethasone on Wednesday. If this happens, they will treat him with a long course of a rela-tively low dose of prednisone to knock out all his chronic GVHD at once.

The plan is that he will remain on his current dose of cyclosporine, the main immunosuppressant, for a month and that after that, if he hasn't had a flare (they're giving 65% odds that he will) he can start tapering over the follow-

166

ing six months. Getting off the cyclosporine and any other immunosuppressants is the biggest issue in allowing him to live as normal a life as possible without being totally paranoid about infections. The kicker is that, if they don't treat his GVHD with these drugs, his immune system won't mature properly and he'll be prone to infections, so the drugs are really a necessary evil.

Another interesting thing is his vitamin supplement. It turns out that MDS patients, for some reason, store iron like mad. In addition, when you get a blood transfusion you get a ton of iron. Dr. W. told us that Brian has now gotten enough iron for two or three lifetimes. He will therefore be taking the "mature" formula vitamins from now on because they are low in iron.

Dr. W. talked to us a lot about what life is going to be like from now on. Brian is now, overall, four times more likely to get cancer than the average person. That's still not a huge risk, but it's there. In particular, he's prone to skin cancer and prostate and colon cancers. He's going to have to be very careful about sun for the rest of his life, which we all should be but few of us are.

The moment of the conference that really got me was when we were talking about returning to normal activities and Dr. W. said, "You've got a lot of life ahead of you, and it's time to start living it." I don't think words can capture what it meant to me to hear that. Just a few short months ago we were wondering if he would have any life ahead of him at all.

Steve Cohen and Jack Sarfaty also had their conferences in the last few days. I'm not sure which one of us is going home first, but we're all going home. I talked to Sharon today, and she's going berserk about getting herself, Steve, their four kids and her mother back to Detroit. Listening to someone else go nuts makes me feel a little better about my own nuttiness.

Dick McKee is still in the hospital and doing OK. We're going to take Suzanne out for ice cream tomorrow night to say goodbye. Don Prichard is plugging along in outpatient, still taking an amazing cocktail of drugs. He's a miracle.

The rest of our day was spent being a tad crazy over packing — Brian has 30 hours less before his departure than we thought. Although I know that going home is a positive milestone, it also feels like a big hurdle. We are suddenly trying to figure out what our contingency plans are if Brian gets sick at home. I'm also feeling very nervous about returning to work and leaving Eve. Last night I had a nightmare where she was taking a nap, and someone was coming over to watch her so I could go out, and I left before the sitter got there and then panicked and tried to go home but couldn't get there. Sound like I'm anxious?

The fact of the matter is that life will never be "normal" again. In the first place, "normal" life entailed not having kids, and that's obviously over. In the second place, Brian is doing well but he's not done with this journey just yet. He's got a lot of medical issues and medications and appointments and tests still ahead of him. In the third place, I don't think I'm the same person I was two years ago. And I'm not sure that's a bad thing.

Eve has been very obliging about all this stress. She has been kind enough to sleep through the night two of the last three nights, and tonight she went to bed 40 minutes early as we get her ready for the time change. Of course, all of this would be greatly helped if her mother could sleep past 5 AM, but hey, it's better than nothing.

The computers are getting packed tomorrow afternoon and won't be rejoining us for over a week, so e-mail updates will be sparse. Don't panic if you don't get floods of e-mail from us in the next week. I'll be getting hives from withdrawal, but I'll manage.

Thank you to all of our friends and family and all the wonderful people on BMT-talk who made this whole time livable. Best of luck to all who battle the beast and courage to all their caregivers. Prayers for all of you whose loved ones have lost the battle. Thanks to those of you who have been our role models through this all. We simply could not have done this without knowing you all are out there. We love you.

naomi

Greetings from Pittsburgh!

Our flight home last Tuesday was very long but relatively uneventful. Eve was pretty fussy. Getting up at 5:30 AM is not her forte, and she barely napped on the plane. Our first flight was late and meals got screwed up. It was the typical, hellish travel experience on our nation's airlines.

We were greeted at the airport by one friend whom we had asked to come help us with luggage and another couple of friends who had simply deduced from our e-mails what flight we must be on and came to surprise us. By the time we landed, we were totally exhausted, so it was nice to have everyone there. The trip really took it out of Brian in particular, although it's hard to tell how much of that was from the trip and how much was actually transplant related. After all, I was pretty darned pooped also.

The last week has been maniacally busy. Brian has been to clinic twice, we bought a second car, we celebrated our 7th wedding anniversary, we've been madly unpacking, we had to restart our cable and newspaper, we had to get our kitty back and get him reacclimated to life with us and with Eve, we had to childproof the house and get gates for stairs and doorways, Eve and I had to have our check-ups and on and on.

In some ways, our homecoming has been anticlimactic. In fact, my first words to the friend who was meeting us at the airport were, "What, no marching band?" It's difficult to discover that, for some reason, the world continued to turn while we were away doing this momentous thing.

We have had some wonderful gestures sent our way, though. Aside from two friends surprising us at the airport, another one stopped by that night, another brought me a zucchini cake (Brian can't have it, but I have no such restrictions, yum!), our neighbors' kids left us welcome home signs on the dining room table the day we arrived, and our Rabbi brought us ice cream. Friends and neighbors arranged to have our house and carpets cleaned before we came home, lent us baby gates and moved breakables off of low shelves in preparation for the newly mobile Ms. Eve.

One of the hardest things about the last week has been trying to explain Brian's current state to people who haven't been following us all along. One person suggested I tell people, "All things considered, he's doing very well," but that's really hard for people to grasp. I've had a number of people tell me they are glad to hear Brian is "better" and it's "smooth sailing from here on in," but of course that's not true. On the other hand, he's not at death's door, either. It's complicated, and it's hard to encapsulate in a quick sentence or two everything you really need to know to explain "How's Brian?"

The week has featured several triumphant returns to our old stomping grounds. Brian was greeted with many friendly smiles, hugs, and "You look like a million bucks!" at the hematologist's office on Thursday. I got similar treatment at Temple on Saturday. It was great to be home and at Temple, since I haven't set foot in a synagogue since well before we left in April. Today, Eve and I went to our family doctor — her for her 15-month check-up and me for my annual oil and lube. It was wonderful to be dealing with a family doctor who is really ours! And, of course, there were hugs all around there, too.

Medically, Brian is doing OK, but not great. He discontinued his beclomethasone on Wednesday and by Friday he had some diarrhea. Monday he actually upchucked his pills for the first time in a long time.

He saw his Pittsburgh doctor for the first time yesterday because she was away last week. Now, I should preface my description of this visit by telling you that she came into the room, said she'd been reading my updates and that, in her words, I'm "cool" and that she thought I had lost weight. So obviously her judgement is seriously impaired. Anyway, it's her feeling that, if Brian's gut GVHD is coming back, it's not coming back fast and she wants to wait and see what happens before doing anything.

So that's the news here. I am starting to "get settled," whatever that means. I start work next Wednesday, which has me fairly stressed out. I think the separation is going to be harder on me than on Eve!

Thanks to everyone who has called or e-mailed the last several days. We are trying to "reconnect" and it's nice to feel like we were missed, at least a little.

naomi

Afterword

"I am the bridge
Over my neck
The people pass from shore to shore
To the happy days in store. . .
And day and night
Night and day, God
This is my prayer
Give me strength their weight to bear."

— Yehoash

Date: Saturday, 23 Oct 1999
Subject: Terror, guilt, and other light topics

As many of you may have already heard, the last three weeks have taken some very wonderful people from this world. Donald Lee Prichard, Jr. died of complications following his bone marrow transplant on October 5. Richard McKee died of CMV pneumonia and graft rejection on October 20. Jack Sarfaty died of an infection in his lungs yesterday, October 22.

I hope what I'm going to say doesn't seem selfish or weird or whatever. I'm scared. I'm really, really, really scared and I don't know what to do with it. We became close with maybe six families through this process and three of the patients are now gone. Someone has to make it, right? Why is this happening?

I also feel guilty. I have allowed myself the hubris of, if not believing Brian was doing well, at least believing he wasn't going to get any worse. And I have allowed myself the hubris of thinking I can point to one reason or another why bad things are happening to others. "He had a bad match." "She had a bad attitude." "His counts were low." But the fact is, if Brian died tomorrow you would all have similar things to say about him. An opportunistic infection could strike tomorrow and he'd be dead by next week. Why is he alive when others aren't? And how do I live with the knowledge of how fast that could change?

Brian's GVHD flared for the second time since coming back to Pittsburgh this week, and they put him back at the beginning of the prednisone treatment he started in September. Others are tapering their cyclosporine, while Brian can't even taper his prednisone. He will be on it at least until the summer, probably longer. He will be that susceptible for that long.

I want it over. I want my life back. I want his life back. I want to be able to talk with our BMT friends about triumph and not loss after loss. I am tired of conversations that begin in hushed tones, "Have you heard from . . ." I am tired of walking downstairs from reading e-mail and telling my husband that we've lost another battle.

I feel like putting my fist into a wall. This situation wasn't fair when it started and it isn't fair in how it's ending for these good people and their families. I feel such an obligation, such a burden, to be the family that makes it. If not, who will live on in memory of those who lost the battle? May their memory be a blessing.

naomi

Brian and I returned today from our one year Long Term Follow-Up visit to the transplant center. Before I give you the news from that, let me bring you up to speed on some things that happened since we last left our hero.

As you may recall, Brian's GVHD flared right after we came home. They put him on prednisone and started a taper, but he flared again. They tried again and he flared again. And a third time. They finally added another immunosuppressant medication, Cellcept®, to the mix, and this did the trick. He's been taking 80 mg of prednisone every other day since January, plus the Cellcept® and the cyclosporine and all his antibiotics, anti-fungals, anti-virals and numerous dietary supplements.

During Brian's second flare, his phosphorous dropped to dangerous levels. It took literally months to figure out what was going on, during which time he had to have frequent six-hour infusions of phosphorous in the clinic to stabilize his counts.

As it turns out, and my high school chemistry teacher would kill me for not noticing this, phosphorous bonds with magnesium and calcium. So every time Brian took his phosphorous supplements at the same time as his calcium and magnesium supplements or with calcium-fortified orange juice, the ions would bond and he would literally pee the whole thing out. It took only about a week after a visit to the endocrinologist to stabilize things.

Brian had his Hickman catheter removed at the beginning of December. I really pushed for this, probably more than Brian did. I told his doctor I didn't like making love to a man with a tube in his chest. This probably wasn't the most tactful thing I could have said, but it worked.

Brian landed at the hospital twice during the last year. Both times it was for bouts of stomach flu that left him dehydrated. While this was scary, IV fluids brought him back to health within 24 hours on both occasions. Both of these episodes occurred entirely outpatient. He hasn't been inpatient since the day he walked out of the hospital last June on day +28. He's been very lucky.

Brian is at about 90% of normal. He takes care of Eve two days a week and is working on his dissertation. He plays racquetball at least once a week and even managed to tear his rotator cuff and fracture his upper arm playing softball. He has completely lost his ability to digest dairy, even with the help of Lactaid®, and no one seems to know when or if that will come back. We joke that he's not lactose intolerant — he's a lactose bigot. But it seems a small price to pay.

Ms. Eve is still the light of my life. She is now two and is just plain amazing. She has an ever-burgeoning vocabulary which, in addition to all the

174

normal two-year-old words, includes "Daddy take pills." Her reality has been altered by this experience, too.

As for me, I returned to work September 1st after almost 18 months away. Leaving Eve was absolutely the hardest thing I have ever done. She was my buddy for 15 months and I felt empty without her. It was also amazing to discover that I still got to be her Mommy, even after I returned to work. The evenings and weekends we spend together are a major love-fest.

My volunteer activities in the world of marrow have grown exponentially. I've coordinated blood drives and marrow drives in Pittsburgh and have been invited to give sermons on our experiences at synagogues. I do lots of fundraising for the Brian Zikmund-Fisher Fund for DR Typing. It continues to grow through individual donations and the occasional charity auction. Jose Carreras did indeed come through with an autograph, on his bow tie, which fetched over $300.

After a year of soul searching, I decided that what I was doing in the area of marrow fundraising and recruitment as a volunteer was plenty. I felt that I could use the skills I had acquired caring for a loved one, battling the health insurance system, creating a fund and generally becoming a resource rather than a victim, in combination with what I was already doing. So, this fall, I will begin classes for my second master's degree, this one leading to certification as an elementary principal.

So now, let's get back to our trip. Going back to the transplant center for the one-year check-up was one of the hardest things I have ever done. Being there was too familiar, and old memories flooded back. I had managed to suppress much of the bad stuff from last year, choosing only to remember some of the fun we had. Being there made me confront the enormity of what we had been through.

Brian got the cleanest bill of health we could reasonably have expected. He still has sub-clinical GVHD of the mouth and skin, but it does not require treatment. He has mild osteoporosis in his spine caused by the prednisone. They predict that that will repair itself once he gets off the steroids. Other than that, he's doing well. His bone marrow is 100% donor cells with no sign of MDS. He will begin tapering his immunosuppressants today and could, if all goes well, be off them by the end of December. On the other hand, we know that these things never seem to progress in a linear fashion.

On this trip, we got to see some of our favorite nurses, our social worker, our volunteer family and our friend Mark. This was a tremendous plus. These people made such a difference in our lives, and it was so nice to feel that we had made an impact on them, too. We took everyone out for a nice dinner to celebrate life. It was a lot of fun.

On our way back, we stopped in Detroit to see Steve and Sharon Cohen. Steve is back to the practice of law. He has had his ups and downs in much the same way that Brian has. He's been on and off medications, and is pretty darn sick of being sick. Aren't we all? We talk to Steve and Sharon about once a month, or whenever we need encouragement or just someone who speaks the same language. It's almost as if Steve and Brian have a pact — I'll hang in if you will.

We saw Carol Slaughterbeck and her family on this trip as well. She is about 18 months post autologous peripheral blood stem-cell transplant for breast cancer and is doing well. She is working and generally of good cheer. We still correspond via e-mail with her and Cliff.

We had dinner one night with Caryn and Richard, another of our "survivor" friends. It was pretty funny because, although I recognized Caryn right away, I didn't recognize Richard at all. You see, he didn't have hair the last time I saw him. Brian looked pretty foreign to them, too.

We also had a bittersweet reunion with Cyndi Prichard. We had dinner and reminisced a little. I still admire her spirit, even though she has clearly been hurt by Don's death. She's still someone I would want by my side if, God forbid, I ever needed a BMT of my own. Along with Brian, of course.

This experience has changed who I am forever. It has also changed my marriage to Brian. We're still struggling through. The mood swings due to prednisone aren't helping either of us. But we will make it, because we aren't willing to give ourselves any other choice.

I look back on the last couple of years and am just plain amazed. Two years ago we were making contingency plans for Brian's death. On this trip, I finally asked the doctor what his life expectancy is. He said it isn't much different from a "normal" person's. What a difference two years makes.

I never thought I'd say this, but when Brian and I are old and grey we'll still be together. And when we look back on our lives, most of what we look back on won't be about bone marrow or blood. We're ready to start living our lives again, at least part of the time.

I thank you for sharing this journey with us and wish you luck with all of your own. I don't know how to end this, so I guess it'll just end. Thanks.

naomi